Ready, Set, Dad: A Complete Pregnancy Guide For Men

Simple Baby Hacks, Practical Advice from Experienced Fathers, and Loving Strategies to Support your Partner

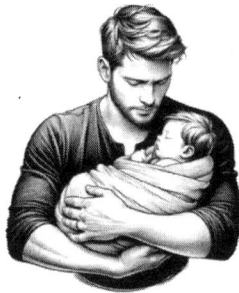

Table of Contents

A Gift for You!

Grab your free workbooks to support your partner and master dad skills now!

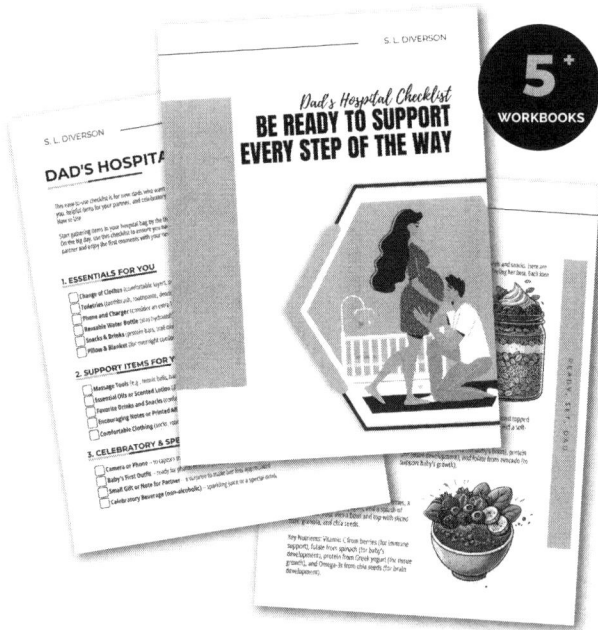

Introduction

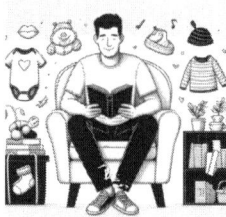

Hey, soon-to-be dads! Ready for the wild roller coaster ride of fatherhood? You're probably thinking, "Fatherhood is a roller coaster? What kind of theme park did I sign up for?" Well, strap in because it's a mix of thrilling, occasionally terrifying, and might make you a tad queasy.

Starting this dad journey might be like tackling a mountain of diapers. Seriously, who knew babies had strong opinions about diaper brands? But fear not; it's not as intimidating as choosing between a gazillion diapers. Sure, there's a bit of fear, but there's also an overload of joy, excitement, and sweet moments that'll make your heart do a happy dance.

Did you know that 9 out of 10 dads actually enjoy changing diapers? I know it sounds like a joke, right? Interestingly, a study by the Centers for Disease Control and Prevention found that 90% of fathers living with their children actively participate in changing diapers (CDC, 2013). Changing a diaper can be more than just a smelly task; it's like a bonding session where you and your little one share a "fragrant" moment.

So, dear soon-to-be dads, let's embark on this adventure together. I'll be your guide, your partner in crime, and we'll face the twists and turns of fatherhood like a dynamic duo.

Fatherhood is like a mixtape of emotions, from the "whoa" moments to the sheer joy of holding your newborn. Each part of this journey is like a note in a song, and trust me, it's going to be your favorite playlist.

Just like a roller coaster has its ups and downs, fatherhood has the highs of seeing your baby's first smile and the lows of wondering if you're doing it right. But hey, it's okay not to have all the answers; the best part is figuring it out while sharing goofy moments with your kid.

Patience is critical in Dad's land. From those late-night diaper changes to the "I don't want to wear that" meltdowns, having patience will be your superhero cape. Celebrate the tiny victories, enjoy the hilarious moments, and savor the everyday chaos—it's more important than you think.

Being a dad is like walking a tightrope. It's about supporting your kid without tripping over your own shoelaces. Find that balance, juggle your responsibilities like a circus act, and create a happy space for both you and your child.

As you dive into this dad adventure, be ready for change. Challenge the outdated ideas about being a dad, forge your own path, and create a home where both parents are the rock stars.

When your kid grows up, it's like passing them the baton. Watching them navigate life is like the grand finale of our roller coaster. Cherish the hilarious memories, share your "dad wisdom," and strut around proudly because you've built an awesome bond.

So, new dads, welcome to the dad roller coaster—a ride full of surprises. Enjoy the craziness, hold onto those hilarious moments, and get ready for the awesome adventure ahead! Strap in, laugh along the way, and brace yourself for the most entertaining ride of your life!

Chapter 1:

The Truth About Morning Sickness

Well, here we are at the starting line of this marathon called fatherhood. The stadium lights are on, and the crowd is going wild. Okay, the "crowd" might just be your partner and your soon-to-be-born baby, but they're definitely rooting for you. And your first hurdle? Morning sickness. But don't worry, champ, we've got this. Let's tackle this beast head-on and dispel some myths about morning sickness along the way.

The Mystery of Morning Sickness: Fact vs. Fiction

Now, about this 'morning' sickness business, it turns out it's more of an 'anytime' sickness. That's right, contrary to its name; morning sickness can strike at dawn, noon, or even under the moon! According to the folks at BabyCenter, some women feel nauseated all day long, while others might find the evenings more challenging. So, dads, keep those crackers handy 24/7 because this party doesn't stick to a schedule!

Picture this: a rollercoaster of queasiness that's not restricted to the crack of dawn. It's an equal-opportunity nausea distributor, ready to make a surprise appearance at any given moment. So, the next time someone insists on calling it "morning" sickness, gently remind them that the party favors include a 24/7 nausea pass, no reservations required.

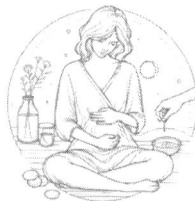

And here's an interesting nugget of information—morning sickness isn't just a human phenomenon. Scientists have observed similar symptoms in animals like dogs and monkeys. So, if you notice your pet dog giving you a sympathetic look while your partner's hugging the toilet bowl, it's not your imagination.

In essence, morning sickness is a misnomer, a linguistic hiccup that deserves a whimsical eye-roll. Whoever named it clearly missed the memo on the whole day-and-night cycle thing. So, brace yourself for a nausea-filled fiesta that follows its own schedule, a party your partner might have unintentionally RSVP'd to—the kind where the pickles can become the unexpected stars, stealing the spotlight at any hour. Welcome to the unpredictable world of morning sickness, where the clock ticks to the beat of its own slightly nauseating drum.

Hormonal Hijinks

Wondering what's behind this queasy carnival? Say hello to hCG, our hormonal headliner! This little hormone, as per Cleveland Clinic and BabyCenter, skyrockets in early pregnancy and brings the nausea along for the ride. It's like hCG throws its own welcome party in your partner's body, and unfortunately, the dress code includes morning sickness. Remember those biology classes you snoozed through? I bet you didn't expect hormones to crash your fatherhood fiesta! This hormone does a lot of good things, like telling your partner's body that she's pregnant and needs to start preparing for a baby. But it's also responsible for making her feel sick.

You see, the levels of hCG rapidly rise during the first trimester. And this dramatic surge is like inviting nausea to come and party in your partner's stomach.

The Good News About Nausea

Now, here's the silver lining. While morning sickness can feel like a cruel joke nature's playing on your partner, it's actually a good sign. According to BabyCenter, studies have shown that morning sickness is associated with a lower risk of miscarriage. So, while your partner battles the belly blues, Mother Nature might just be giving you a thumbs up, signaling all is well on the baby front! Another study published in JAMA Internal Medicine found that women who experienced nausea and vomiting were 50-75% less likely to experience a miscarriage.

So, while your partner may be cursing her relentless nausea, it's actually a reassuring sign that her pregnancy is on track. It's as if Mother Nature's saying, "Hey, I know you're feeling lousy, but it's all part of the plan."

Now, this doesn't mean you should be alarmed if your partner isn't experiencing morning sickness. Every pregnancy is unique, much like every dad's reaction to assembling a baby crib (you'll get there, I promise).

So there you have it, the lowdown on morning sickness. It's not just for mornings; mischievous hormones cause it, and while it's not exactly fun, it's a sign that your partner's body is doing exactly what it needs to do.

And remember, you're in this together. So, when your partner dashes to the bathroom at the whiff of coffee, your job is to be there for her. Hold back her hair, rub her back, and remind her she's a warrior. Because even though it doesn't feel like it right now, morning sickness is just a tiny part of this incredible journey you're both on. And I promise you, it's all worth it in the end.

It's not just about being there for the baby's milestones; it's also about being there for your partner through every burp, belch, and bout of nausea. Because that's what being a dad is all about. It's about stepping up, showing up, and cleaning up, even when the going gets tough. And trust me, the rewards are worth every minute. But more on that later. For now, let's keep tackling these hurdles one at a time.

How to Support Your Partner Through Morning Sickness

Hey, champ! Now that we've cracked the morning sickness code, it's time to gear up with some superhero moves to help your partner power through it. Yup, you heard me right. While you can't zap away the queasy, there are a bunch of things you can do to make this ride a bit less rocky. And guess what? Your part is more than that of a passive observer; you have the opportunity to be an encouraging ally—the Batman to her morning sickness mayhem. So, let's break it down, superhero style!

First things first, realize you're not on the sidelines for this one. You're in the game, my friend. From being the midnight pickle supplier to nailing the art of sympathetic nods, you have what it takes to be the unsung hero. It's time to flip through the partner support handbook— we're about to show morning sickness that it's no match for your dynamic duo. Get ready for some laughs, a few groans, and a whole lot of superhero antics. It's go time!

The Power of Peppermint Tea

Picture this. It's a chilly morning. Your partner wakes up, her face a shade paler than usual. You know what's coming. She's about to make a sprint to the bathroom. But wait, what's that you're holding? A steaming cup of peppermint tea. You hand it to her, she takes a sip, and there it is—that sigh of relief.

Peppermint tea isn't just a refreshing morning brew. It's a natural remedy for nausea. Its minty aroma soothes the stomach and can help ease the queasiness caused by morning sickness. So, why not turn tea-making into your morning ritual? It's a small act, but it shows your partner that you're there for her, ready to tackle the day and its challenges together.

The Ginger Root Rescue

Now, let's talk ginger. No, not the redhead down the street, the root. Ginger has been a trusted ally against nausea for centuries. In fact, studies show that ginger can significantly reduce nausea and vomiting during pregnancy. What to Expect sings praises of ginger's nausea-nixing powers. Whether it's ginger ale that actually contains real ginger or those zesty ginger candies, this root is your secret weapon in the anti-nausea arsenal. Who knew that a simple spice could be the superhero in the saga of stomach serenity?

So, how can you incorporate ginger into your partner's diet? Well, ginger tea is a good start. But there's more: Ginger biscuits, ginger candies, even ginger-infused water. There's a world of ginger possibilities out there. But remember, too much of a good thing can be, well, not so good. So, please keep it to a reasonable amount, about one gram of ginger per day.

The Crackers-In-Bed Hack

Now, this next hack might sound a bit odd, but bear with me—crackers in bed. Yes, you read that right. Keeping a stash of crackers on the nightstand has saved many pregnant women from the clutches of morning sickness.

You see, an empty stomach can aggravate morning sickness. But who feels like eating when they're feeling nauseous? That's where crackers come in. They're bland, easy to eat, and can help settle the stomach. So, before your partner even thinks about getting out of bed, hand her a few crackers to nibble on.

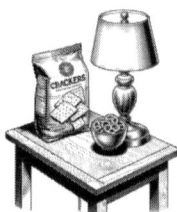

And there you have it, the trifecta of morning sickness remedies—peppermint tea, ginger, and crackers. But remember, everyone's different. What works for one person might not work for another. So, don't be discouraged if the first remedy you try isn't a hit. Keep trying, supporting, and showing your partner that she's not going through this alone. Because that's what this is all about. It's not just about finding the perfect remedy; it's about showing up, day in and day out, and reminding your partner that you're in this together, come morning sickness or high water.

And remember, while morning sickness might feel like it's lasting an eternity, it's only a small part of the pregnancy. It doesn't define your partner's pregnancy, and it certainly doesn't determine your journey into fatherhood. It's just one hurdle in the race, and you're more than equipped to handle it. So, keep your head high, your peppermint tea steaming, and your ginger at the ready. This is just the beginning, champ. And you're doing great.

What Not to Say to a Woman Experiencing Morning Sickness

The "It's All in Your Head" Blunder

Let's kick things off with a classic mistake. Picture this: your partner, green-faced and grimacing, is clutching her stomach. In a misguided attempt to provide reassurance, you tell her, "It's all in your head." Oops, you've just stepped on a verbal landmine.

You see, morning sickness isn't some phantom symptom. It isn't a figment of her imagination. It's as real as the baby bump that'll soon be part of your daily life. Telling her it's all in her head? It's like telling her that her feelings and physical discomfort don't matter. Not exactly the message you want to send, right?

Instead, try acknowledging her struggle. A simple "I know you're feeling terrible, and I'm here for you" can go a long way in making her feel seen and supported. Remember, you're her partner, not her psychiatrist. Validate her feelings; don't analyze them.

The "At Least You're Not..." Faux Pas

Now, onto our next verbal slip-up. The "At least you're not..." statement. You tell her, "At least you're not vomiting all day," or "At least you're not bedridden." You might think you're helping her see the silver lining, but guess what? You're not.

Comparing her experience to someone else's doesn't make her feel better. It makes her feel like her suffering isn't valid. Every woman's pregnancy experience is unique. Some experience mild symptoms, some severe. Some might even sail through without a bout of nausea. But that doesn't make her struggle any less real.

So, ditch the comparisons. Instead, let her know that you understand she's struggling. You can't walk in her shoes, but you can walk alongside her. And that's what she needs right now—not comparisons, but compassion.

The "You're Overreacting" Misstep

Finally, let's address the "You're overreacting" comment. Here's the thing. Pregnancy is a profound, life-altering experience. It's like being strapped into a rollercoaster seat without an exit button. And guess what? Morning sickness is one of the scariest loops in the ride.

Telling her she's overreacting is like telling her she's wrong for feeling the way she does. But there's no right or wrong way to react to morning sickness. She's not being dramatic or seeking attention. She's coping with a spiral of changes happening inside her body.

Instead of dismissing her feelings, ask her how you can support her. Maybe she needs a comforting word, a loving hug, or just the reassurance that you're there for her.

And there you have it. Navigating the morning sickness conversation doesn't have to be a minefield. With a bit of empathy, understanding, and a whole lot of patience, you can provide the emotional support she needs. And remember, the goal isn't to fix everything. It's to let her know that she's not alone. That you're in this together. Now, and for all the loops, turns, and thrilling drops that lie ahead on this rollercoaster ride into parenthood.

Morning Sickness Survival Kit: What to Include

Alright, champ, we've made it this far. We've debunked myths and discussed dos and don'ts, and now, we're about to put together your secret weapon: the morning sickness survival kit. Think of it as your Batman utility belt, but instead of grappling hooks and smoke pellets, you have ginger candies and extra pillows. Ready to start packing? Let's do it.

The Hydration Heroes: Water and Sports Drinks

First up, we have the hydration heroes. Now, you might be thinking, "Water? Really? I thought this was going to be some groundbreaking stuff!" Well, stick with me here. When your partner is dealing with morning sickness, keeping her hydrated is crucial. Between the nausea and the vomiting, she might get dehydrated, which is a no-go during pregnancy.

But why stop at water? Sports drinks are another great addition to the survival kit. They're not just for athletes, you know. Sports drinks contain electrolytes, which help replenish the body's water levels and keep nausea at bay. Plus, they come in different flavors, which can help break the monotony of plain water. So, pack a few bottles of water and sports drinks, and you're good to go.

The Snack Saviors: Crackers and Pretzels

Next, we have the snack saviors. Now, remember when we talked about the crackers-in-bed hack? Well, it's time to put that into action. Crackers are a fantastic snack to keep on hand. They're bland, easy to eat, and can help settle the stomach. But why stop at crackers? Pretzels are another great option. They're salty, crunchy, and just as easy on the stomach as crackers.

So, keep a stash of these snack saviors in your survival kit. They're perfect for those times when your partner needs a quick nibble to keep the nausea at bay. Plus, they're portable, which means she can have them on the go. Talk about a win-win!

The Soothing Sidekicks: Ginger Candies and Peppermint Gum

Now, let's move on to the soothing sidekicks. We've already sung the praises of ginger and peppermint, so let's put them to work. Ginger candies are a great way to keep the benefits of ginger on hand. They're sweet and spicy and can help soothe the stomach. Plus, they're easy to carry around, making them an excellent option for those unexpected waves of nausea.

Peppermint gum is another fantastic addition to the survival kit. It's refreshing, easy to chew, and can help ease queasiness. Plus, it's a great way to freshen up after a bout of morning sickness.

The Comfort Companions: Extra Pillows and Cozy Blankets

Last but not least, we have the comfort companions. Now, I know what you're thinking. "Pillows and blankets? This is a survival kit, not a slumber party!" Well, trust me on this one. When your partner is dealing with morning sickness, comfort is key. And what's more comforting than a soft pillow and a cozy blanket?

Extra pillows can help prop her up, making her feel more comfortable. A cozy blanket can provide warmth and comfort, helping her relax. Plus, it's a nice way to show her that you care.

And there you go, your morning sickness survival kit. It's not just about the items you pack; it's about the thought and care that goes into it. It's about showing your partner that you're there for her, ready to face this challenge with her. So, pack that kit, champ. You're well on your way to acing this fatherhood thing.

Breakdown of Pregnancy By Weeks

- **First Trimester**

  Weeks 1-4: This is like the starting point based on your partner's last period. The baby-making magic happens around week 2, and a tiny egg moves into the womb.

  Weeks 5-8: Now things get interesting. The baby's first heartbeat kicks in, transforming from an embryo into a tiny human. Around week 5, according to Mayo Clinic, the levels of hCG hormone increase, leading to significant changes in your partner's body. The embryo starts to develop three distinct layers, each of which will form different parts of your baby, like the heart, bones, and kidneys. By the end of week 8, your tiny human might be just about half an inch long—that's about half the diameter of a U.S. quarter!

  Weeks 9-12: Organs start to shape up, and the baby looks more like a little person. Good news—the risk of anything going wrong goes down.

- **Second Trimester**

  Weeks 13-16: The tough early days may ease up. Morning sickness might chill out, and your partner might feel the baby moving. The Cleveland Clinic tells us that this is when the pregnancy starts to show. The fetus begins to make movements, such as sucking its thumb. Imagine, by the end of month four, your baby is as big as an avocado!

  Weeks 17-20: Time for a cool ultrasound where you might find out if it's a boy or a girl. The baby's bones start to harden. Your partner might start feeling the baby move, which feels like a flutter at first. The baby's skin is still thin, but it starts to put on some fat, and by the end of the fifth month, your baby is about

9 to 10 inches long and weighs around a pound. Quite the growth spurt!

Weeks 21-24: Lungs are getting ready, and the baby's skin is less see-through. Your partner might start to really look pregnant.

- **Third Trimester**

Weeks 25-28: Heading into the home stretch! The Cleveland Clinic informs us that from weeks 25 to 28, the fetus's skin gets plumper and less wrinkled. By the end of the seventh month, your baby could be 14 to 15 inches long, weighing between 2 and 3 pounds. In the following weeks, your baby will be maturing and is preparing for the big debut.

Weeks 29-32: Baby's bones are good to go, but still gaining some weight. Get ready for more belly; your partner might start feeling "practice" contractions.

Weeks 33-36: Baby's getting ready to come out and may flip into a head-down position. The lungs are almost there. Your partner might start feeling a bit more uncomfortable.

Weeks 37-40+: Full-term! The baby's pretty much cooked and could arrive anytime now. Mom might show signs of labor, but it's okay if things go a bit past the due date.

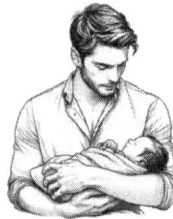

Chapter 2:

Trimester Breakdown—What to Expect

Have you ever been on a road trip with no map or GPS—just the open road and a sense of adventure? That's what the first trimester feels like. It's a winding road of surprising turns, unexpected pit stops, and breathtaking views. And just like any road trip, having a co-pilot makes it all the more bearable. So, grab your metaphorical map, fasten your seatbelt, and let's hit the road.

The First Trimester: A Roller Coaster of Changes

In the first trimester, your partner might feel really tired and possibly nauseous. It's like she's on a long hike with an invisible backpack. Her body is also going through a transformation, with her breasts becoming tender and heavier. Oh, and don't be surprised if she dashes to the bathroom more often—her growing uterus is putting pressure on her bladder!

The Pregnancy Test Plot Twist

Picture this: Your partner hands you a small plastic stick with two tiny lines. You're holding a positive pregnancy test. Welcome to the plot twist of your life. This tiny device, not much bigger than a pen, has just delivered life-altering news—you're going to be a dad.

This moment might be filled with all kinds of emotions—exhilaration, fear, joy, disbelief. You might feel like your heart is about to burst out of your chest like a jack-in-the-box. It's okay. These feelings are perfectly normal. Take a deep breath, let it sink in, and allow the reality to wash over you.

The Hormonal Hurricane

Once the initial shock wears off, you'll step into the eye of the hormonal hurricane. Remember, your partner's body is now a baby-making factory working 24/7. Her hormones are the diligent workers ensuring everything runs smoothly.

One of the key players is human chorionic gonadotropin (hCG), the team leader. Its job is to keep the pregnancy going and make sure other hormones are produced. It's like the factory boss ensuring all operations proceed without a hitch.

Another hormone on the production line is progesterone. This hormone helps the uterus prepare for the baby, thickening the lining to create a nurturing environment. Think of it as the interior designer, fluffing up the pillows and ensuring everything is comfy and cozy.

With all these hormones flooding her system, your partner may experience mood swings, nausea, and fatigue. She's not being moody or lazy; she's simply responding to the hormonal changes in her body. So, when she cries at a diaper commercial or naps at noon, remember to be patient and understanding.

The Fatigue Fog

Remember those all-nighters you pulled in college, surviving solely on caffeine and adrenaline? Imagine feeling like that but without the caffeine or adrenaline to keep you going. That's what the fatigue in the first trimester feels like.

Your partner is growing a new life, and that's exhausting work. Her body is diverting energy to the baby, leaving her feeling drained. So, if she wants to nap or go to bed early, let her. She's not being lazy; she's listening to her body's needs.

This is where you can step in as a supportive partner. Help out with household chores, make dinner, or simply offer a comforting massage. Small acts of kindness can go a long way in helping her navigate the fatigue fog.

As a first-time dad, the first trimester can feel like a windstorm of changes. But remember, you're not just a eyewitness. You're an proactive participant in this journey. So, show up, step up, and embrace the road ahead. Because this is just the beginning of your incredible adventure into fatherhood.

The Second Trimester: From Bump to Baby Kicks

As you enter the second trimester, things might start to stabilize. Your partner might feel less nauseous and more emotionally balanced, like finding a calm spot in the midst of a storm. Physically, she might experience swelling in her feet and ankles, so maybe it's time to try those foot massages! And remember, if she's dealing with nasal congestion, it's just another quirky part of pregnancy.

The Baby Bump Debut

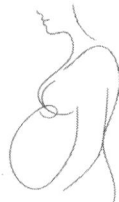

Alright, dad-to-be, let's cruise into the second trimester, a stage often referred to as the 'honeymoon period' of pregnancy. And one of the highlights? The grand appearance of the baby bump. It's like the red carpet moment at an awards show, where your baby decides it's time to let the world know they're on board.

Up until this point, your partner's pregnancy might have felt somewhat abstract, something you knew was happening but couldn't quite see. But now, as her belly begins to round out and the maternity clothes make their way into her wardrobe, things start to get real. This is your baby making their presence known.

As the bump grows, you might be amazed at the transformation your partner's body is undergoing. It's a visual reminder of the remarkable process of creating new life. You may even find yourself talking to the baby bump, a way of bonding with your unseen little one.

The Kicks and Wiggles Waltz

When you thought the second trimester couldn't get any more exciting, along comes another milestone—the baby's first movements. It's like your baby is hosting a private dance party, and your partner is the exclusive guest.

These initial sensations, often described as flutters or wiggles, might be complex for your partner to distinguish at first. It's a feeling she's never experienced before, like having a tiny butterfly fluttering around in her belly. But as the weeks pass, those flutters will grow stronger, turning into unmistakable kicks and jabs.

Imagine this. You're lounging on the couch, your hand resting on your partner's belly, and then it happens. You feel a tiny thump against your hand. That's your little one saying, "Hello, Dad! I'm here!" It's a magical moment, a tangible sign of the life you both have created.

The "Is That a Foot?" Phenomenon

Now, as these dance-offs in the womb become more frequent and stronger, you and your partner might find yourselves playing a guessing game—the "Is that a foot?" phenomenon. Was that little lump a foot, a hand, or maybe an elbow? It's as if your baby is playing hide and seek, giving you little clues about their position.

It's also pretty common for babies to have active and quiet periods. They're just like us, after all. Sometimes, they're up and ready to boogie; other times, they're all about the chill vibes. So, don't worry if there are periods of quiet. Your baby is likely just catching some Z's.

Welcome to the second trimester, where the concept of having a baby becomes more tangible. The baby bump, the first kicks, the games of guess-the-body-part. These are the moments that make the ride worthwhile. So, soak it all in, dad-to-be. These are the days you'll look back on with a heart full of love and a smile on your face.

The Third Trimester: The Final Countdown

The third trimester is like the final act of a play. Your partner may feel more tired and uncomfortable, and yes, a bit more forgetful. As the due date approaches, it's normal for her to worry about labor. Her body is preparing for the grand finale, with the baby placing pressure on her lungs, making it harder to breathe" (Health Hive, n.d.).

The Nesting Instinct Invasion

Alright, future dad, we've reached the final stretch. The third trimester. It's like the last mile of a marathon, the last piece of a jigsaw puzzle, the last level of a video game. And one of the first signs that you're in the homestretch? The nesting instinct.

Now, you might be thinking, "Nesting? Isn't that something birds do?" Well, yes, but in this context, nesting refers to the urge pregnant women feel to clean, organize, and prepare their home for the baby's arrival. Nesting is like an internal call to get everything ready for the baby, and it kicks in towards the end. And as for not seeing her feet, it's just a sign that your baby is growing and making its presence known" (Health Hive, n.d.; Grünebaum, 2019).

You might find your partner cleaning out closets, organizing baby clothes, or setting up the nursery at 2 a.m. It's like she's been taken over by a hyper-organized, super-motivated alter ego. And your role in this? Be her sidekick. Help her with the heavy lifting, run those late-night errands, and lend a listening ear when she's deciding between baby blue or sky blue for the nursery walls.

The "Where Are My Feet?" Dilemma

Now, let's talk about the elephant in the room. Or should I say the baby bump in the room? As your partner's belly grows, she might start to experience the "Where are my feet?" dilemma. It's like her belly has taken center stage, pushing everything else out of view.

She might struggle with simple tasks like tying her shoes or picking up something from the floor. It's like her body's playing a game of hide and seek, and her feet are always hiding. Your job? Step in and lend a hand when she needs it. Help her put on her shoes, pick up that dropped pen, and reassure her that her feet are still there, just hiding behind her beautiful baby bump.

The Braxton Hicks False Alarms

Finally, let's address those pesky Braxton Hicks contractions. Imagine them as the body's fire drill, preparing for the real event. These contractions are the body's way of preparing for labor, flexing and relaxing those uterine muscles.

However, these "practice contractions" can sometimes feel pretty darn close to the real thing, leading to some false-alarm trips to the hospital. It's like having a pop quiz when you were expecting the final exam.

The key to distinguishing Braxton Hicks from real contractions lies in their frequency and intensity. While real contractions grow more frequent and intense over time, Braxton Hicks tends to be irregular and often disappear with movement or a change in position.

Tell your partner to try lying on her left side, use pillows for support, and practice good sleep habits. If heartburn and indigestion bother her, eating small meals, avoiding greasy foods, and not lying down right after meals can help. And for the all-too-common morning sickness, eating several small meals throughout the day rather than three large ones can be beneficial" (Office on Women's Health, n.d.).

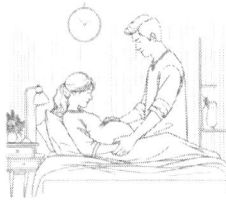

So, there you have it. The final lap of the pregnancy marathon. It's a time of intense anticipation, preparation, and, yes, a bit of anxiety. But remember, you're not a mere spectator in this process. You're a key player. Your role is to be there for your partner, lending your strength, patience, and unwavering support on this final stretch to the finish line.

Trimester Comparison: The Highs and the Lows

The Energy Peaks and Valleys

Imagine a mountain range. Majestic peaks rise, only to descend into deep valleys. The same is true for energy levels during pregnancy. They ebb and flow, creating a unique landscape that shifts with each trimester.

In the first trimester, energy levels may drop, making your partner feel like she's perpetually climbing a steep hill. This is due to hormonal changes and the sheer amount of work her body is doing to create a new life. Don't be surprised if she needs more rest than usual.

The second trimester often brings a much-needed energy boost, similar to reaching a plateau where the view is fantastic, and the climb isn't as steep. With morning sickness usually tapering off, your partner may find herself feeling more like her old self.

The third trimester, however, can feel like a downhill trek. As your partner's body grows heavier with the baby's weight, she might feel more tired and need more rest. This is normal and is her body's way of preparing for the physical demands of childbirth.

The Mood Swing Merry-Go-Round

Welcome to the mood swing merry-go-round, a ride that's as unpredictable as it is inevitable. One minute, your partner might laugh at a joke; the next, she might cry over a sentimental commercial.

In the first trimester, hormonal changes can send her emotions on a wild ride. Joy, anxiety, excitement, fear—it's a veritable whirlwind. Your role here is to provide a stable grounding, a calm place amidst the storm.

The second trimester usually offers a more even-keeled ride. As hormone levels stabilize, so do emotions. This is often a period of relative calm and enjoyment as your partner adjusts to the reality of pregnancy.

But hold on tight because the third trimester can bring another round of emotional ups and downs. As the reality of impending parenthood sets in, it's normal for her to feel a mix of anticipation, excitement, and perhaps a bit of nervousness.

The Anticipation vs. Anxiety Tug-of-War

The journey of pregnancy is a dance between anticipation and anxiety. It's a tug-of-war that plays out over nine months.

The first trimester is often filled with anticipation. There's the thrill of the positive pregnancy test, the excitement of sharing the news, and the joy of imagining what your little one will look like. But it can also bring anxiety—concerns about miscarriage, worries about health, and fears about becoming a parent.

During the second trimester, anticipation usually wins the tug-of-war. With the risk of miscarriage significantly reduced and the reality of the baby bump, most couples feel a sense of excitement and joy.

In the third trimester, however, you can see anxiety pulling back. As the due date approaches, it's natural for both of you to have concerns about labor, delivery, and the realities of caring for a newborn.

Just remember, it's okay to feel a mix of emotions. Pregnancy is a profound life transition, and it's expected to have worries. The key is to communicate openly, support each other, and know that it's okay to seek help if the anxiety feels overwhelming.

So here we are, standing at the edge of an incredible new frontier. The trimesters have come and gone, each bringing its unique blend of highs and lows, challenges and triumphs. You've navigated the ebbs and flows of energy, ridden the mood swing merry-go-round, and played tug-of-war with anticipation and anxiety. You've been there, supporting your partner every step of the way.

As we turn the page, let's remember that this isn't just about surviving the trimesters. It's about thriving. It's about embracing the changes, weathering the storms, and celebrating the calm moments. Because the journey to fatherhood is more than a series of trimesters. It's an experience that will transform, challenge, and ultimately enrich you in ways you never imagined. Now, let's continue our adventure.

Chapter 3:

Embracing Your Role—The Unsung Hero of Pregnancy

Picture this: you're standing on a stage, lights blinding you, the audience buzzing with anticipation. Suddenly, the curtain lifts, revealing you in a superhero suit. You strike a pose, and the crowd erupts into applause. It feels good, doesn't it? Well, my friend, in the world of pregnancy, you're not just an expectant dad; you're a superhero. Now, let's find out what your powers are.

Embracing Your Role: Beyond the Provider Stereotype

The Emotional Support Superhero

So, here's your first superpower: emotional support. Imagine it as a glowing orb of empathy, kindness, and understanding. It's the power to tune into your partner's feelings, provide comfort during tough times, and celebrate the joys of pregnancy together.

Picture a difficult day: your partner's hormones are on a rollercoaster ride, she's exhausted, and morning sickness is rearing its ugly head. As her emotional support superhero, your powers can make a world of difference. You're the reassuring voice that tells her it's okay to rest, the comforting presence that soothes her worries, and the understanding partner who doesn't get upset when dinner plans are canceled at the last minute because the smell of pasta makes her nauseous.

As her emotional support superhero, your understanding and empathy are crucial. According to a study published in BMC Pregnancy and

Childbirth, women greatly value the social support they receive during pregnancy, significantly impacting their emotional well-being. Your role as a reassuring and understanding partner aligns with this research, underscoring the importance of your support during this journey.

You might not be able to whisk away her discomfort with a wave of a magic wand, but your emotional support is a superpower in its own right. It's the force that helps her feel understood, loved, and less alone during this challenging yet exciting time.

The Household Chore Champion

Next up, we have your household chore champion power. This is the ability to step up your game around the house, taking on tasks to ease your partner's load. Think of it like a super-speed power, enabling you to whizz around the house, tackling chores efficiently and gracefully. MountainStar Medical Group (2023) emphasizes the role of partners in ensuring the well-being of expectant mothers by sharing household responsibilities. By easing the physical load, you demonstrate teamwork and shared commitment, which is vital during pregnancy.

Let's set the scene. Your partner comes home after a tiring day, her back aching and her feet swollen. She walks into the house, expecting to see a pile of dirty dishes and laundry. But what's this? The dishes are done, the laundry is folded, and the house smells of fresh coffee. You, my friend, have just used your household chore champion power.

Taking on more chores doesn't just lighten your partner's physical load. It also shows her that you're a team, sharing responsibilities and supporting each other. So, roll up your sleeves, put on your favorite tunes, and let your Household Chore Champion power shine.

The Pregnancy Education Enthusiast

Now, let's reveal your third superpower: The pregnancy education enthusiast. This superpower enables you to delve deeply into the world of pregnancy knowledge. You'll understand the changes occurring in your partner's body and your baby's development. Organizations like

Tommy's, which concentrate on pregnancy health, emphasize the significance of partners educating themselves about these transformations. Fortunately, by reading this book, you've already started gathering valuable insights about pregnancy. You're well ahead in the game! Your proactive learning equips you to offer effective support to your partner during this transformative journey.

Imagine this: Your partner is worried about a new pregnancy symptom. She's searched online, but the flood of information only makes her more anxious. Enter you, armed with knowledge from reputable sources, ready to dispel myths and provide accurate information. You're not just easing her worries but also becoming a hands-on contributor in the pregnancy, understanding the process and what your partner is going through.

Becoming a pregnancy education enthusiast means doing your homework. Read books, attend prenatal classes, follow expert blogs, or even download pregnancy apps. The more you learn, the more you can support your partner and connect with your upcoming journey into fatherhood.

So, there you have it, your superpowers for the pregnancy journey. You're the emotional support superhero, the household chore champion, and the pregnancy education enthusiast. But remember, every superhero needs a sidekick. In this case, your sidekick is empathy, patience, and a sense of humor. Use them wisely, and remember, you're not just a supporting character in this story; you're sharing the lead role with your partner, ready to step into the adventure of parenthood together.

Ways to Participate Actively During Pregnancy

The Prenatal Class Companion

Alright, future dad, it's time to head back to school—no, not algebra class or that dreaded history lecture. We're talking about prenatal classes—a treasure trove of knowledge for soon-to-be parents. And you, my friend, are not just a silent observer. You're the prenatal class companion, actively participating in this learning journey.

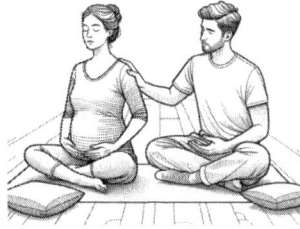

So, what does being a prenatal class companion entail? Well, it's about more than just showing up. It's about engaging, asking questions, and soaking up knowledge like a sponge. This aligns with advice from Dr. Ramos-Jensen, as reported by KSL.com, who underscores the importance of attending prenatal appointments together.

Picture this: You're sitting in a cozy room, surrounded by other expectant couples. The instructor is demonstrating a breathing technique. With your undivided attention, you are practicing alongside your partner, encouraging her, and committing the steps to memory.

And it's not just about the class sessions. It's about bringing that knowledge home, practicing the techniques, discussing what you've learned, and applying it to your journey. You're not just a companion in class but also a companion in learning, growing, and preparing for parenthood.

The Baby Gear Guru

Next on the agenda, it's time to channel your inner gadget geek. Welcome to your role as the baby gear guru. From strollers and car seats to baby monitors and diaper bins, there's a whole universe of baby gear to explore.

Think of yourself as an explorer navigating through the dense jungle of baby products. Your tools? Research, reviews, and a keen eye for safety and practicality.

Imagine this scenario: You're standing in a baby store, a labyrinth of products stretching out before you. Armed with your research, you expertly navigate through the aisles, selecting a car seat with top safety ratings, a stroller that's easy to fold and carry, and a baby monitor with excellent reviews.

But your role doesn't end there. Once the gear is home, you're on assembly duty. And no, it's different than when you tried assembling a bookshelf and ended up with a lopsided mess. You're taking your time, following instructions, and ensuring everything is safe and secure for your little one.

Through this process, you're not just becoming a baby gear guru but also a protector, creating a safe, comfortable environment for your baby to thrive in.

The Birth Plan Partner

Finally, let's talk about your role as the birth plan partner. A birth plan is a blueprint for labor and delivery, outlining your partner's preferences for things like pain relief, delivery positions, and immediate postpartum care. And you, my friend, are an integral part of this planning process.

Think about it this way: You and your partner are architects, designing a plan for one of the most significant events of your lives. You're discussing, researching, and making decisions together.

Imagine you and your partner sitting together with a blank sheet of paper. You discuss what she wants, share your thoughts, and create a plan that respects her choices and makes her comfortable. If she's into placenta encapsulation (making pills from the placenta), add it to the birth plan.

What is placenta encapsulation? It's when they dry out and put the placenta into pills. Some people believe it helps after giving birth. To do this, talk to a specialist before your due date, inform the hospital staff and add it to your birth plan with the paperwork. Starting this talk early is important to match the hospital rules and make everything go smoothly.

Working on a birth plan together and understanding your partner's preferences for labor are key aspects of being the birth plan partner. This collaborative approach, as recommended by health professionals like Dr. Ramos-Jensen on KSL.com, ensures both partners' voices are heard and respected, thus creating a supportive and empowering environment for birth.

But it's not just about creating the plan; it's also about advocating for it. When the big day arrives, you're there by her side, ensuring her wishes are respected and that she feels supported and heard.

Being a birth plan partner means being an ally, a supporter, and a voice for your partner during a profound and transformative moment in her life.

And there you have it. As a prenatal class companion, you're engaging in the learning process. As a baby gear guru, you're navigating through the world of baby products. And as a birth plan partner, you're advocating for your partner's wishes during labor and delivery.

Embrace these roles. Immerse yourself in them. By doing so, you're actively participating in the pregnancy, connecting with your partner, and preparing for the incredible adventure of fatherhood. You're not just a spectator; you're on the field, playing the game and making a difference. So, go ahead, step into your roles, and let your superpowers shine.

How to Be a Supportive Partner During Medical Appointments

The Note-Taking Ninja

Alright, dad-to-be, you've got your superpowers, your cape is crisp, and your alter-ego is ready. Now, it's time to step into the role of the note-taking ninja. Medical appointments can feel like a ton of information, with medical jargon flying left and right, tests being ordered, and advice being given. Amidst all this, your partner might feel overwhelmed or forget to ask crucial questions. That's where you swoop in, notepad at the ready.

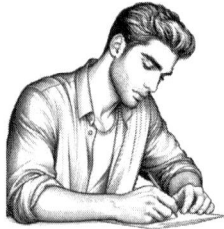

As the note-taking ninja, you're there to jot down the important details. The doctor mentioned a strange-sounding term? You write it down for later research. A date for an ultrasound was set? You've got it noted. Does a particular symptom need monitoring? It's in your notes.

But remember, note-taking isn't just about scribbling down medical terms. It's about capturing the essence of the appointment. Did the doctor mention any concerns? What were the positive highlights? What steps need to be taken before the next visit? Your notes are a tangible record of the appointment that you and your partner can refer to later.

The Question-Asking Advocate

Next up, let's talk about your role as the question-asking advocate. Medical appointments can sometimes feel one-sided, with the doctor imparting information and your partner nodding along. But remember, these appointments are not just for receiving information; they're also for asking questions. And that's where your advocacy comes in.

As the question-asking advocate, you're there to ensure your partner's concerns are heard. If she's too shy to ask or if she forgets, you've got her back. From understanding medical terms to clarifying the doctor's advice, no question is too small or unimportant.

Keep in mind your role as an advocate goes beyond just asking questions. It's about fostering an open dialogue with the healthcare provider. It's about ensuring your partner feels heard, understood, and cared for. So, raise your hand, clear your throat, and let those questions fly.

Hand-Holding Hero

Finally, let's not forget one of the most important roles—the hand-holding hero. No, this isn't just about literally holding your partner's hand (though that's important too). It's about providing emotional support during these medical visits.

Medical appointments can be nerve-wracking. Your partner might need emotional reassurance, whether it's anxiety over test results or just general nerves. As the Hand-Holding Hero, your power lies in your ability to provide comfort. A reassuring hand squeeze, a confident nod, a shared joke to lighten the mood—these are your tools as the hand-holding hero.

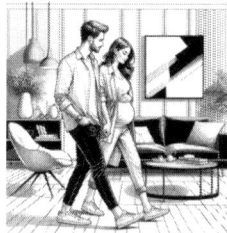

Remember, your presence at appointments is more than just physical. It's a source of comfort, a pillar of support, and a reminder that she's not alone in this. You're there with her, for better or worse, in sickness and health. So, squeeze her hand, look her in the eye, and remind her that you're in this together every step of the way.

So, future dad, grab your notepad, prepare your questions, and get ready to hold hands like a pro. You're not just an attendee in these medical appointments; you're an committed participant. You're the note-taking ninja, the question-asking advocate, and the hand-holding hero. By embracing these roles, you're showing your partner that you're there for her in every way possible. You're showing her that you're not just her partner but her superhero.

Why Your Emotional Support Matters

The Hormonal Harmony Impact

Picture this. You're in a ballet theater, watching a performance. Each dancer moves flawlessly, their steps perfectly timed, creating a breathtaking spectacle of harmony. Now, think of this ballet as your partner's hormonal system during pregnancy. Each hormone performs its role in sync, maintaining a delicate balance.

During pregnancy, your partner's body is juggling a surge of hormones. This hormonal upheaval not only influences her physical state but also her emotional well-being. Mood swings, anxiety, weepiness—they're all part of the hormonal performance.

And this is where your emotional support enters the stage. By providing a steady stream of reassurance, understanding, and empathy, you can help maintain this delicate hormonal harmony. It's like being the conductor of the orchestra, assisting each musician in—or, in this case, hormone—performing at its best.

The Bonding Benefit

Now, let's shift our attention to a different stage—the stage of bonding. Yes, bonding isn't just a post-birth phenomenon. It begins during pregnancy itself, and your emotional support plays a starring role.

When you show your partner emotional support, you're not just helping her; you're also building a connection with your unborn baby. Each comforting touch, each shared laugh, each word of encouragement echoes in the womb. It's like your love and support are forming an invisible bond, connecting you, your partner, and your baby.

This bonding isn't just emotionally beneficial; it's also scientifically significant. Research shows that babies can recognize voices heard in the womb once they're born. So, each time you talk to the baby bump or read a bedtime story, you're forming a connection, a familiar thread that your baby will recognize in the outside world.

The Stress-Reducing Ripple Effect

Finally, let's dive into the sea of stress reduction. Picture it as a calm sea, with your emotional support creating ripples of relaxation across its surface.

Pregnancy can be a stressful time. These stressors can pile up like a stack of unwashed dishes, from physical discomfort to the anxiety of impending parenthood. And we all know that stress isn't a great houseguest. It overstays its welcome and creates a mess.

Your emotional support can help evict this unwanted guest. By lending a listening ear, offering comforting words, or simply being there for your partner, you can help reduce her stress levels. It's like you're creating ripples in the sea of stress, calming the waves and bringing a sense of tranquility.

And this stress reduction isn't just beneficial for your partner; it's also good for the baby. Studies show that high stress levels during pregnancy can impact the baby's development. So, by reducing your partner's stress, you're helping her and creating a healthier environment for your baby.

So, that sums it up. Your emotional support isn't just a sweet gesture; it's a necessity, a force of good. It aids hormonal harmony, fosters bonding, and reduces stress. It's like your love and care have a ripple effect, spreading positivity and well-being in its wake.

So, step into your role as the unsung hero of pregnancy. Be the steady hand that offers support, the comforting voice that reassures, and the loving partner who is there every step of the way. Because your emotional support matters—to your partner, your baby, and the incredible adventure of parenthood that lies ahead.

And as the curtain falls on this chapter, remember, you're not just a audience member in this pregnancy but an active participant. You're the emotional support superhero, the household chore champion, the pregnancy education enthusiast, the prenatal class companion, the baby gear guru, the birth plan partner, the note-taking ninja, the question-asking advocate, and the hand-holding hero. You're a key player on this team, and your role is crucial, valued, and appreciated.

As we turn the page and explore the next stage of this adventure, remember—you're a superhero in this story. And every superhero, no matter how powerful, has one thing in common —a heart that cares. So, wear your cape with pride, future dad. The journey continues, and the best is yet to come.

Chapter 4:

Navigating the Emotional Rapids—Understanding and Supporting Your Partner's Feelings

Pop quiz, soon-to-be dad! What do you get when you mix a dash of joy, a sprinkle of anxiety, a dollop of irritability, and a generous helping of tearfulness? No, it's not a recipe for disaster—it's the emotional cocktail of pregnancy. As your partner's hormones dance the cha-cha-cha inside her body, her emotions might feel like they're riding the world's fastest roller coaster. But fear not because you're about to become an expert in understanding and navigating this emotional terrain. So, buckle up, and let's dive right in!

The Emotional Roller Coaster: Hormones and Emotions

The Tearful Tidal Waves

Ever seen a grown woman cry over a TV commercial? Or a slightly overcooked dinner? Welcome to the world of tearful tidal waves. Blame it on the hormones! The surge in pregnancy hormones like progesterone and estrogen can lead to significant emotional fluctuations. According to BMC Pregnancy and Childbirth, the hormonal changes during pregnancy can result in heightened emotions, leading to episodes of tearfulness or irritability. Understanding that these reactions are normal and part of the hormonal changes is important.

It's like her tear ducts have a mind of their own, ready to unleash a flood at the slightest trigger. She might cry over things that would normally barely register on her emotional radar. It's important to remember that she's not being overly sensitive or dramatic; she's just riding the hormonal waves.

So, what can you do? Be her emotional buoy. Keep a stash of tissues handy, offer comforting words, or simply hold her hand. Sometimes, silence is the best support you can offer.

The Irritability Icebergs

The next stop on our emotional roller coaster ride is Irritability Icebergs. Remember the placid lake of patience your partner used to be? Well, pregnancy hormones can turn that lake into a stormy sea, with icebergs of irritability lurking beneath the surface.

A forgotten chore, a casual comment, or even a minor inconvenience can trigger an irritable response. It's like walking on eggshells around a grumpy cat. But don't take it personally. It's not about you; it's the hormones pulling the strings.

Your superhero power here is patience. Try to stay calm, even if her irritability pushes your buttons. Keep communication open, and if things get heated, take a break to cool down. Remember, this isn't the new normal; it's just a temporary detour on the pregnancy journey.

The Joyful Jolts

We've talked about the tears and the irritability, but let's remember the joyful jolts. Pregnancy isn't just a hormonal thunderstorm; it's also a rainbow of joy and excitement. Feeling the baby kick, seeing the baby bump grow, planning the nursery—these are moments of pure, unfiltered joy.

Seeing your partner's face light up at the first flutter of baby movements or her excitement at fitting into maternity clothes—these are the moments that make the hormonal roller coaster worth the ride.

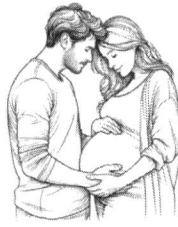

Your role in these moments? Be an integral partaker in her joy. Share in her excitement, celebrate the milestones, and create happy memories together. Pregnancy is a journey of highs and lows; the joyful jolts are the scenic viewpoints you don't want to miss.

Alright, dad-to-be, you're now equipped with the knowledge to understand and navigate the emotional roller coaster of pregnancy. You're ready to face the tearful tidal waves, steer clear of the irritability icebergs, and ride the joyful jolts. But remember, your journey isn't over yet. We still have plenty to explore in the realm of emotional support. So, keep your superhero cape on, and let's continue this adventure together!

How to Help Your Partner Navigate Emotional Changes

The Empathy Exercise

Let's kick things off with the empathy exercise. Now, you may wonder, "What is the empathy exercise?" Well, it's not about doing push-ups or lifting weights. It's about flexing your emotional muscles, particularly the one that allows you to feel and understand what your partner is experiencing. As found in a qualitative study by BMC Pregnancy and Childbirth (Al-Mutawtah et al., 2023), partners who show understanding and empathy can greatly alleviate the emotional burden of pregnancy. It's about more than just listening; it's about validating your partner's feelings and providing comfort in response to their emotional state.

Imagine stepping into your partner's shoes for a moment. Consider the changes she's going through: the hormonal tornado, the physical transformations, the anticipation, and the anxiety. It's a lot to handle. By practicing empathy, you're acknowledging her feelings, validating her experiences, and letting her know that she's not alone in this.

But remember, empathy isn't just about understanding; it's about showing that understanding. A comforting touch, a sympathetic nod, a reassuring word—these are the ways you can express your empathy. It's about turning your understanding into action and creating a supportive environment where your partner feels seen, heard, and loved.

The Patience Practice

Next up is the patience practice. Now, patience is a virtue, and during pregnancy, it's a strength. As your partner navigates the emotional rapids of pregnancy, there might be moments when her mood flips faster than a pancake on a hot griddle. One moment, she's all smiles; the next, she's in tears, and you're left wondering what just happened.

This is where your patience comes into play. It's about accepting these mood swings as part of the pregnancy package, not as a reflection of your partner's character. It's about biting your tongue when you feel unfairly snapped at and extending a hug instead of a harsh word.

Remember, practicing patience isn't about being a doormat; it's about choosing your battles and understanding that this emotional turbulence is temporary. It's about standing steady in the face of the storm, knowing that clear skies are approaching.

The Communication Code

Finally, let's crack the communication code. Open, honest, and respectful communication is the cornerstone of any relationship, and during pregnancy, it's as essential as prenatal vitamins. As your partner experiences a cascade of changes, having a clear line of communication can help both of you navigate this new terrain.

Now, communication isn't just about talking; it's also about listening. It's about giving your partner space to express her feelings, fears, and hopes without interruption or judgment. It's about asking open-ended questions that invite her to share more rather than shutting down the conversation with yes-or-no queries.

But remember, the communication code isn't a one-way street. It's also about expressing your feelings, sharing your concerns, and actively participating in the conversation. It's about building a dialogue where both of you feel heard, respected, and understood.

There's the rundown for you. The empathy exercise, the patience practice, the communication code—these are your tools to help your partner navigate her emotional changes during pregnancy. It's not about fixing things or finding solutions; it's about providing support, understanding, and love. It's about creating a safe harbor where she can weather the storm, knowing that you're sailing the ship together.

Avoiding Common Mistakes in Emotional Support

The Problem-Solving Pitfall

Picture this: your partner comes to you teary-eyed, sharing how overwhelmed she feels with the changes in her body, the emotional turmoil, and the anxiety about becoming a mom. You, wanting to make her feel better, immediately jump into problem-solving mode, offering solutions, suggesting remedies, and devising plans. But rather than making her feel better, it just seems to add to her frustration.

Welcome to the Problem-Solving Pitfall. It's a common mistake many of us make, thinking that the best way to support our loved ones is by fixing their problems. But here's the thing: sometimes, people don't need solutions; they just need to be heard.

According to Tommy's, a UK-based pregnancy charity, sometimes the best support you can give is simply to be there, offering a listening ear and a reassuring hug. Avoid minimizing or dismissing her feelings, as this can make her feel misunderstood or isolated. Your partner is experiencing a twister of changes, and sometimes, she might need to vent to express her feelings without worrying about finding solutions. So, rather than rushing to fix things, try simply listening, acknowledging her feelings, and offering comfort.

The Minimizing Mistake

Next up is the Minimizing Mistake, a misstep that can unintentionally hurt your partner's feelings and make her feel misunderstood. Let's say your partner is sharing her concerns about labor, and you respond with, "Don't worry, women have been doing this for centuries." While your intention might be to reassure her, it can come across as minimizing or dismissing her feelings.

Remember, what might seem like a minor concern to you might be a big deal for her. Dismissing or minimizing her fears and concerns can make her feel like her feelings are not valid or important.

Instead, try to validate her feelings. Even if you don't fully understand her concerns, let her know that it's okay to feel the way she does and that you're there to support her. A simple "I can see why you're worried, and I'm here for you" can go a long way in making her feel understood and supported.

The Unsolicited Advice Slip-up

Last but not least, we have the Unsolicited Advice Slip-up. Imagine your partner complaining about her swollen feet after a long day, and you immediately chiming in with advice on what she should or shouldn't do. While your intention might be to help, offering unsolicited advice can sometimes make her feel like you're not really listening to her but rather waiting for your turn to speak.

When your partner shares her struggles, she might not be looking for advice. Sometimes, she might just want a sympathetic ear, a comforting embrace, or a simple "that sounds really tough."

If you feel like she could use some advice, ask her first if she wants it. A simple "I have some thoughts on this; would you like to hear them?" shows that you respect her feelings and her autonomy.

In conclusion, being a supportive partner isn't about fixing problems, minimizing concerns, or offering unsolicited advice. It's about being there, listening, validating feelings, and offering support. By avoiding these common mistakes, you can provide the emotional support your partner needs during this transformative time. And remember, you're not just supporting her; you're also building a solid foundation for your journey into parenthood.

The Power of Empathetic Listening

The "Just Listen" Lesson

You know that feeling when you're so engrossed in a movie that you forget about the popcorn in your hand? That's what empathetic listening is like. It's about being fully present and completely absorbed in what your partner is saying. It's not about planning your response or thinking about dinner. It's about giving her your undivided attention. A study by Tommy's emphasizes the importance of partners being present and acknowledging the emotional experiences of pregnant women. This includes offering physical comfort and verbal reassurance that validate her feelings and experiences during this time.

Imagine this situation: Your partner is sharing her worries about becoming a mom. Instead of interrupting with your thoughts or solutions, you stay silent, maintaining eye contact and nodding to show you're listening. You're giving her space to express herself, vent, and let it all out. That's the power of the "just listen" lesson.

The "Validate Feelings" Victory

Now, let's move on to the next stage of empathetic listening—the "Validate Feelings" victory. Remember when you were a kid and you won that gold star in school? And how it made you glow with pride? Validation is like that gold star. It's a recognition of your partner's feelings, confirming that what she's experiencing is real and important.

For example, your partner is upset because her favorite jeans no longer fit her growing baby bump. Instead of dismissing it as a trivial issue, you validate her feelings. You acknowledge that it's hard to see her body changing so rapidly and that it's okay to feel a sense of loss. You're not just saying, "I hear you," you're saying, "I understand, and your feelings are valid."

The "Offer Comfort" Commandment

Finally, we arrive at the "offer comfort" commandment. Think of comfort as a warm blanket on a chilly night. After opening up about her feelings, it's soothing, reassuring, and just what your partner needs.

Offering comfort comes in many forms. It could be a hug, a reassuring smile, a comforting word, or a gentle squeeze of the hand. It's about showing your partner that you're there for her and that she's not alone in her feelings.

For instance, if your partner is feeling anxious about labor, you offer comfort. You reassure her that she's strong, that she can do this, and that you'll be there with her every step of the way. You're not trying to fix or dismiss her anxiety; you're comforting her, offering a safe and supportive space to express her worries.

Thats the gist of it, future dad. You've unlocked the power of empathetic listening. You've learned to listen, to validate feelings, and to offer comfort. These aren't just skills; they're tools you can use to support your partner during her pregnancy. They're ways you can connect with her, understand her, and grow together as you prepare for the arrival of your little one. So, keep practicing, keep listening, and keep validating. Your journey into fatherhood is just getting started.

As we leave the terrain of emotional changes and empathetic listening, gear up for the next stage of this exciting expedition. Up next, we dive into the fascinating world of pregnancy's physical changes. From understanding what's happening inside her body to knowing how to offer help and support, get ready to explore, learn, and grow as a soon-to-be dad.

Chapter 5:

Navigating the Uncharted Waters— Understanding Labor Stages

Let's face it: future dad, labor, and birth are like navigating uncharted waters. It's a voyage into the unknown, filled with anticipation, excitement, and a fair bit of anxiety. But fear not, my fellow explorer, for we're about to map out these waters and equip you with the knowledge to confidently sail through them. So, grab your compass, hoist the sails, and let's set out on this enlightening adventure!

Understanding the Stages of Labor

Labor is like a marathon, not a sprint. It's a process that unfolds gradually, marked by different stages and phases. Knowing what to expect can help you support your partner effectively during labor. Let's start our exploration by understanding the stages of labor.

Labor is typically divided into three main stages. The first stage involves the onset of labor until the cervix is fully dilated to 10 centimeters. This stage itself has two phases: early labor, where the cervix dilates to about 4 to 6 centimeters, and active labor, where dilation progresses from 4 to 6 centimeters to about 7 to 8 centimeters. Active labor is characterized by more intense and frequent contractions, coming about every three to four minutes apart.

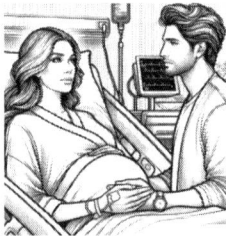

Early Labor

Think of early labor as the calm before the storm. It's the initial stage of labor, often the longest but least intense. Your partner might not even realize she's in labor at this point, mistaking the contractions for a mild backache or menstrual cramps.

Your partner's cervix gradually dilates to about 4 to 6 centimeters. This stage can last from six to twelve hours, with contractions becoming stronger and more frequent over time. But don't worry; the contractions are usually moderate and manageable during early labor, spaced about five minutes apart as labor progresses. This information comes straight from the experts at What to Expect, who provide a comprehensive look at early labor signs and symptoms.

During early labor, her cervix starts to soften, thin out, and dilate. Contractions at this stage are usually far apart, lasting 30 to 45 seconds and giving plenty of rest in between. It's like nature's way of easing her into the labor process.

Active Labor

Now, we're getting into the thick of it. The calm waters of early labor give way to the choppier waves of active labor. Contractions become longer, stronger, and closer together. It's like the drumroll before the grand finale, increasing intensity and frequency.

During active labor, your partner's cervix dilates from 3 centimeters to about 7 centimeters. This is usually the stage where most women head to the hospital or birthing center. The intensity of contractions can make it harder for your partner to talk or laugh through them, unlike early labor.

Transition Phase

Hold on tight because we're now entering the most intense part of labor—the transition phase. It's like reaching the peak of a roller coaster ride right before the exhilarating drop. Contractions are usually very strong, lasting 60 to 90 seconds and coming about two to three minutes apart.

During this phase, your partner's cervix dilates from 7 centimeters to a full 10 centimeters. Transition is often the most challenging part of labor, characterized by intense discomfort and firm pressure in the lower back and rectum. But remember, it's also the shortest phase.

Pushing and Birth

In a hospital setting, childbirth can vary significantly, particularly if your partner has an epidural. This decision impacts her sensation of contractions, with the epidural potentially numbing the pain. When this is the case, the medical team becomes instrumental, alerting her to each contraction's onset and guiding her on when to push.

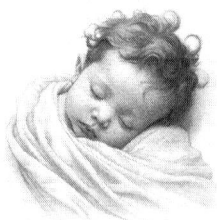

The pushing phase can vary in duration, ranging from a few minutes to several hours. It's a demanding test of endurance, akin to the final, intense moments of a marathon or a tug of war. During this time, your partner will be guided by her instincts or the medical team's instructions.

Then, in an instant, as your baby is born, the pain and anticipation give way to an indescribable wave of emotions. All at once, there's an overwhelming sense of intense love and happiness. Words fall short in capturing this moment. In this instant, as you hold your newborn, the reality sets in: you are now a dad!

This moment marks the beginning of a new chapter. The journey of labor, filled with its highs and lows, transitions into a lifetime of parenting. The challenges and joys of raising a child await, each day bringing new experiences, learning, and unconditional love. Welcome to fatherhood – a journey unlike any other.

Delivery of the Placenta

Wait, we're not done just yet. After your baby is born, there's one more stage to go—the delivery of the placenta, also known as the afterbirth. This is like the cool-down period after a strenuous workout.

Contractions continue after birth but are much less painful. These contractions help separate the placenta from the uterus and push it out. This usually happens within 5 to 30 minutes after birth. Once the placenta is delivered, the labor process is officially complete.

Some experts, including those at What to Expect, highlight the two to three hours after the delivery of the placenta as a critical time for both bonding and monitoring for any abnormal bleeding. This period is not only essential for the medical team to ensure everything is proceeding normally post-delivery, but it's also an ideal opportunity for mom and newborn to engage in skin-to-skin contact. Skin-to-skin contact offers numerous benefits: it helps regulate the baby's body temperature, heart rate, and breathing, and it can also encourage a more successful start to breastfeeding. Additionally, this intimate contact releases oxytocin, often referred to as the 'love hormone,' which can enhance maternal bonding and reduce stress for both the mother and the baby.

Voilà, a clear breakdown of the labor stages. Understanding these stages can help you provide your partner with the support she needs during labor. It's like having a map for the uncharted waters of labor and birth, guiding you through the voyage and helping you confidently navigate the waves. So, keep this knowledge at hand, future dad, as you prepare to embark on the incredible journey of childbirth.

Routine Baby Exams At The Hospital

Shortly after being born in the hospital, newborn babies undergo a series of routine exams and assessments to ensure their health and well-being. These evaluations are crucial for identifying any potential issues and providing early intervention if needed.

The initial assessment includes the Apgar score, which assesses the baby's heart rate, respiratory rate, muscle tone, reflexes, and skin color at 1 and 5 minutes after birth. A thorough physical examination is conducted, measuring the baby's head circumference, weight, length, and overall appearance. Vital signs like heart rate, respiratory rate, and temperature are closely monitored.

Healthcare providers also examine the baby's skin for rashes, birthmarks, or other anomalies, and they may check the eyes for any signs of infection. Hearing tests might be performed to detect hearing impairments, and a heel prick blood test screens for various metabolic and genetic disorders.

Additionally, the healthcare team assesses the baby's reflexes, respiratory and heart health, umbilical cord stump, and feeding capabilities. They inquire about bowel movements and urination patterns and may administer initial vaccinations, such as the hepatitis B vaccine, if necessary.

These comprehensive examinations and screenings are vital for ensuring the well-being of newborns and providing timely care and intervention when required, varying slightly based on hospital protocols and the baby's individual health status.

Daddy Duties Shortly After Birth

As a new dad, there are several important responsibilities you'll have shortly after your baby's birth in the hospital or birthing place. First and foremost, offer emotional support and comfort to both your partner and your newborn. Holding your baby, speaking to them in a soothing manner, and being present are all ways to establish a strong bond from the start.

If your partner has undergone a c-section, it's especially important to consider participating in skin-to-skin contact with your baby if the hospital encourages it. This practice not only helps regulate your baby's temperature and reduces stress but also fosters that crucial initial connection between you and your newborn.

Feeding A Newborn

When it comes to taking care of your newborn, feeding is a crucial aspect. Whether your partner is breastfeeding or you're using formula, you can actively participate by helping with positioning and latching if needed. It's essential to follow a feeding schedule for your baby, as newborns typically require a feeding every 2-3 hours.

In addition to feeding, ensure you maintain a comfortable and safe environment for your little one. Regularly changing diapers is crucial to keep your baby clean and comfortable. Moreover, pay attention to cues of hunger, like rooting or fussiness, outside of the scheduled feeds.

Swaddling A Newborn

Make the most of the expertise of healthcare professionals while you have access to them. They can provide valuable guidance on how to correctly swaddle your newborn baby. Keep in mind that once you leave the healthcare setting, you'll be responsible for swaddling your baby on your own.

Mastering the art of swaddling can prove highly advantageous, as it can promote your baby's sense of security and improve their sleep. Additionally, remember to burp your baby after each feeding to alleviate any discomfort caused by gas.

Bathing A Newborn

Bathing your baby for the first time in the hospital can be a special moment. Be gentle and follow the guidance of the nursing staff if you're unsure. Spend quality time bonding with your newborn through conversation, eye contact, and skin-to-skin contact when possible.

Finally, don't hesitate to ask questions and seek advice from hospital staff, especially if this is your first child. They can provide valuable insights into newborn care, safe sleep practices, and more. Building a strong support network can make this journey smoother for both you and your new family.

Embrace these early responsibilities as a father, and cherish the precious moments you'll create with your newborn during these first few days in the hospital. Your support and care are essential for both your baby and your partner as you embark on this incredible journey of parenthood together.

The Lowdown on C-Sections and Epidurals

Reasons for a C-Section

Alright, future dad, let's chat about C-sections, also known as Cesarean deliveries. Picture it as an alternative route to your destination—not the scenic route you initially planned, but a shortcut that gets you where you need to go safely and effectively.

Sometimes, C-sections are planned in advance due to known conditions, like if the baby is breech (positioned feet or bottom first) or if the mom has a medical condition like high blood pressure. Other times, they're decided during labor if complications arise, such as the baby showing signs of distress or labor not progressing despite strong contractions.

Remember, the aim is a safe delivery for both mom and baby. If a C-section is the safest route, it's the best one, even if it wasn't part of the original travel plan.

The Procedure of a C-Section

Now, let's get a sneak peek into the operating room. A C-section is a surgical procedure, but it's a routine one, performed countless times by skilled medical professionals.

Your partner will receive anesthesia—usually a spinal block or an epidural—that numbs the lower half of her body. She'll be awake but won't feel any pain—just some pressure or tugging sensation.

A screen will be set up so she won't see the actual surgery. The doctor then makes an incision in the lower abdomen and uterus, and voila, your baby is lifted out into the world. The entire procedure takes about 45 minutes to an hour, with the actual delivery of the baby taking only a few minutes.

Understanding Epidurals

Next, let's demystify epidurals, the superheroes of pain management during labor, and learn how this incredible ally is administered. Picture an epidural as your partner's loyal sidekick, ready to come to the rescue when the contractions become overwhelming. Administered through a thin tube (or catheter) inserted into the epidural space in the lower spine, an epidural delivers anesthesia that numbs the lower part of the body, significantly alleviating the discomfort of contractions. The beauty of an epidural lies in its ability to provide pain relief while keeping your partner awake and alert during the delivery process.

Now, let's delve into the process of how an epidural is administered. Your partner will simply roll her back as much as she can over her large belly and must remain extraordinarily still. This stillness is crucial to ensure accurate placement of the epidural catheter.

When considering the timing for an epidural, it's generally advised to wait until labor is well-established. This typically means waiting until the cervix is dilated to at least 4 to 5 centimeters, and contractions are occurring regularly. Opting for an epidural too early may potentially slow down labor progress, while waiting too long might make it less effective or more challenging to administer. Nonetheless, it's important to remember that each labor experience is unique, so it's essential to collaborate closely with the healthcare team to determine the most suitable timing for an epidural based on your partner's individual circumstances.

Risks and Benefits of Epidurals

As with any superhero, epidurals have their strengths and weaknesses. On the positive side, they are highly effective at relieving labor pain, allowing your partner to rest during a prolonged labor, and they can be topped up if needed. However, epidurals can also present side effects, such as a drop in blood pressure, itching, nausea, or post-birth headaches. They might slow down labor and potentially make pushing more difficult. It's important to note that for some women, epidurals may not work effectively. If this happens, the medical team will guide you through the next steps and discuss alternative medication options for pain relief. Weighing the benefits against the risks is crucial in making an informed decision that suits both of you.

Recovery From a C-Section

Now, let's talk recovery. After a C-section, your partner is going to need some extra TLC. C-sections are major abdominal surgery, and recovery takes time.

In the hospital, she'll receive pain relief and will be encouraged to get up and move around as soon as she's able. Once home, she'll need to take it easy. This is where you come into play. Help with the baby, do the housework, prepare meals, and remind her to take her pain medication and rest.

Remember, every woman's recovery journey is different. It's important for your partner to listen to her body, to rest when she needs to, and to seek medical advice if she's concerned about her recovery.

So, future dad, you're now equipped with knowledge about C-sections and epidurals. Keep this information in your dad-toolbox. It'll help you understand the process, support your partner, and make informed decisions about your baby's birth. Whether your baby arrives via the scenic route or the shortcut, the destination remains the same—the start of your new life as a family. And let me tell you, no matter how you get there, it's a pretty spectacular place to be.

The Role of a Doula: Should You Get One?

The Doula Difference: What a Doula Does

Imagine having a supportive, knowledgeable guide by your side during the grand adventure of labor and birth. Someone who's been down this road before, knows the twists and turns, and can provide comfort, guidance, and assurance. That future dad is a doula.

A doula is a skilled expert offering ongoing emotional, physical, and informational assistance to a mother before, during, and shortly after giving birth. Picture a doula like a sherpa, guiding your partner through the Himalayas of labor, helping her climb the peaks and navigate the valleys.

She's there to offer soothing words during intense contractions, suggest comfortable positions, and provide reassurance. A doula complements the medical team, focusing on your partner's emotional well-being and comfort.

The Doula Dividends: Benefits of Having a Doula

Now, you might be wondering, "Do we really need a doula?" It's a fair question. After all, you plan to be there, offering support and encouragement. So, why bring a doula into the picture?

Research suggests that having a doula can have several benefits. It's like adding an extra layer of support, enhancing the birth experience for both of you. Studies have shown that having a doula can lead to shorter labor, reduced need for pain medication, fewer C-sections, and increased satisfaction with the birth experience.

But the benefits aren't just for your partner. A doula can also help you. She can guide you in supporting your partner, suggest ways for you to be involved, and provide reassurance. It's like having a coach guiding you through the game, helping you play your best.

Doula Detective: How to Find a Doula

So, you're considering getting a doula. Great! But where do you start? Consider it like a treasure hunt, and you're on the quest for the perfect doula.

Start by asking for recommendations from friends, family, or your healthcare provider. You can also look for certified doulas through reputable organizations. Once you have a few names, set up interviews. Remember, finding a doula who matches well with you and your partner, someone you both feel comfortable with is essential.

Doula Dialogues: Questions to Ask When Hiring a Doula

During the interview, consider yourself an investigative journalist, asking insightful questions to get to the heart of the matter. You want to understand her philosophy about birth, her approach to supporting moms and partners, and her availability around your due date.

Ask about her training, experience, and certification. Find out what services she offers. Does she provide prenatal and postpartum visits? Can she assist with breastfeeding? What's her fee, and what does it cover?

Also, discuss hypothetical situations. How would she help if labor is long and difficult? How would she support your partner if plans change, like a sudden need for a C-section? These questions can give you a sense of how she would handle different scenarios.

So, there you have it, future dad. A walkthrough of what a doula does, the benefits of having one, how to find one, and what to ask during the interview. Understanding the role of a doula can help you make an informed decision about whether to include one in your childbirth team.

Remember, whether or not to hire a doula is a personal decision based on your partner's comfort, your budget, and your birth preferences. The goal is to create a birth environment where your partner feels supported, empowered, and at ease. Whether that includes a doula is entirely up to you.

As we wrap up our exploration of labor, remember this: labor is not just a process; it's an experience. It's the final stretch of the pregnancy marathon, the culmination of months of anticipation, and the gateway to parenthood.

As we move forward, we'll continue to equip you with the knowledge, tools, and strategies to navigate the incredible adventure of becoming a dad. So, keep your eyes on the horizon, future dad. The voyage continues, and the best is yet to come!

Make a Difference with Your Review

Unlock the Power of Fatherhood Insight

"Being a dad is about more than just providing; it's about guiding with a heart full of love." - Unknown

Hey there, amazing soon-to-be dads! Did you know that by helping others, we often end up helping ourselves? That's right, it's like a boomerang of goodness! And speaking of goodness, I've got a little favor to ask.

Ever thought about how you could make a big impact on another dad's life, even if you never meet them? Well, here's your chance. Imagine a fellow dad out there, just like you were before – excited, a bit nervous, and eagerly looking for guidance on this wild ride of fatherhood.

Our mission at S. L. Diverson is simple: we want to make the journey of fatherhood easier and more enjoyable for every dad out there. Everything we do is driven by this goal. But to reach all these amazing dads, we need your help.

You see, most people do judge a book by its cover - and its reviews. So, here's my heartfelt request on behalf of a dad-to-be out there you've never met:

Could you please take a moment to leave a review for "Ready, Set, Dad: A Complete Pregnancy Guide for Men"?

Your review doesn't cost a dime, takes less than a minute, but can change another dad's life forever. Your words could help…

…one more dad feel confident in his new role.

…one more partner support their expecting spouse.

…one more family bond over the miracle of life.

…one more father create unforgettable memories.

…one more dream of a happy family become a reality.

To spread this joy and make a real difference, just scan the QR code below to leave your review:

If the thought of helping a fellow dad brings a smile to your face, then you're exactly who we're looking for. Welcome to the club - you're one of the amazing ones.

I can't wait to guide you through more fatherhood hacks, tips, and heartwarming stories in the upcoming chapters.

Thank you from the bottom of my heart for your generosity and spirit. Now, let's dive back into the adventure of fatherhood!

Your biggest fan,

S. L. Diverson

PS - Fun fact: Sharing is caring! If you think this book is a treasure trove for dads, why not share it with a dad-to-be? Your recommendation could be the greatest gift they receive.

Chapter 6:

The Invisible Umbilical Cord—
Bonding With Your Unborn Baby

Picture this. You're at a rock concert, jamming to the music, feeling the rhythm course through your body. Now, imagine that concert is happening inside your partner's belly, with your unborn baby as the adoring fan. Every word you speak, every song you sing, every story you tell—they're all part of this prenatal performance that your baby is soaking up. Welcome to the world of in-utero bonding, where you get to connect with your baby before they're even born.

Why is this important? Just like a band needs to rehearse before the big concert, you need to practice your parenting skills before the big arrival. And guess what? The rehearsal starts now. By actively bonding with your unborn baby, you're not just forming a connection with them; you're also stepping into your role as a dad. So, grab your metaphorical guitar, warm up your vocal cords, and start this prenatal concert!

How Dads Can Connect with Their Unborn Child

Attending Prenatal Appointments

Think of prenatal appointments as backstage passes to the most exclusive concert in town. Engaging in prenatal appointments and classes is crucial for bonding with your unborn child (Mayo Clinic, n.d.). These sessions offer a window into your baby's development and prepare you for parenthood. These visits offer a sneak peek into your baby's world, giving you a chance to hear their heartbeat (the sweetest melody you'll ever hear) and see them on the ultrasound (the best music video ever).

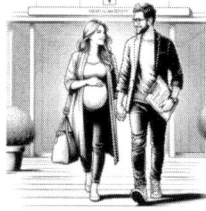

Being there for these appointments means more than just holding your partner's hand. It's an opportunity to ask questions, understand what's happening, and actively participate in the pregnancy. It's like you're part of the road crew, setting up the stage for the big concert. So, mark these dates on your calendar and make sure you're there, front and center.

Reading to the Baby Bump

Ever tried singing a lullaby to the baby bump? It might sound strange, but your unborn baby can hear sounds from the outside world. Around the 23rd week of pregnancy, your baby's ears are well-developed, and they start responding to sounds.

So why not make the most of this by reading to the baby bump? Pick a children's book, a poem, or even a chapter from your favorite novel and read it out loud. This not only helps you bond with your baby but also gets them used to the sound of your voice.

Just imagine the day when you read the same story to your newborn, and they recognize it from the womb. It's like an inside joke between you two, a shared secret from your prenatal bonding days.

Responding to Baby's Movements

Around the middle of the second trimester, your partner will start feeling the baby's movements. At first, they might feel like gentle flutters, but as your baby grows, these will evolve into noticeable kicks and nudges. From 18 to 24 weeks, your unborn baby becomes sensitive to touch, a perfect opportunity for bonding (Dad Gold, n.d.). Gentle interactions can lead to responses from your baby, strengthening your connection.

Respond to these movements by gently rubbing the baby bump or talking to your baby. This interaction can stimulate more movements, creating a unique bonding experience. It's like a silent conversation between you and your unborn baby, a connection that transcends words.

Participating in a Prenatal Class

Prenatal classes are not just for moms-to-be. They're also for dads-to-be like you. These classes can help you understand what's happening during pregnancy, what to expect during labor and birth, and how to care for your newborn.

But more than that, attending a prenatal class shows your commitment to being an involved dad. It's a declaration that you're not just a observer in this pregnancy; you're an engaged contributor, eager to learn, and ready to support your partner every step of the way.

So, future dad, are you ready to rock this prenatal concert? Remember, bonding with your unborn baby isn't just a feel-good activity; it's a stepping stone to fatherhood. It's about forming a connection that begins in the womb and lasts a lifetime. It's about rehearsing your role as a dad, tuning your instruments, and getting ready for the grand performance. So, step onto that stage, grab that microphone, and let the prenatal performance begin!

Fun Activities to Bond with Your Baby Bump

Playing Music for the Baby

You've probably heard of the Mozart effect, the theory that listening to classical music can boost a baby's brain development. While it's not scientifically proven, letting your baby listen to some soothing tunes doesn't hurt.

Think of it as your baby's first concert right in the womb. You can play gentle music, classical symphonies, or even your favorite rock ballads. The genre doesn't matter. What matters is the rhythm, the melody, and the vibration of sound waves that your baby can feel.

Playing music to your unborn baby can be a delightful bonding activity. Setting aside daily music time can familiarize them with various sounds (Dad Gold, n.d.). Make this a ritual. Every night, before bedtime, let your baby listen to a song. It's a moment of peace, a lullaby before dreams, a bond woven with notes and rhythms.

Creating a Baby Bump Cast

Have you ever wanted to freeze a moment in time? To capture it in its raw, unfiltered essence? Creating a baby bump cast allows you to do just that. It's a 3D snapshot of your partner's pregnant form, a keepsake that you can cherish for years to come.

This activity is not just about the end product but also the process. It's about slathering your partner's belly with casting material, laughing at the mess, and marveling at the miracle of her pregnant form. It's a tangible way to celebrate the pregnancy, to appreciate the journey, and to create a memory that will last a lifetime.

Taking Weekly Baby Bump Photos

In the age of selfies and social media, why not start a photo journal of the baby bump? It's like a visual diary, a timeline of growth, a testament to the miracle of life. Writing a letter to your unborn baby and documenting the pregnancy journey can create lasting memories (Mayo Clinic Staff, n.d.). These activities are emotionally significant.

Start from the first trimester and take weekly photos of the baby bump. You can have fun with this. Use props, make funny faces, or simply capture candid moments. It's not about creating perfect shots but about documenting the transformation, the anticipation, the love that grows along with the baby bump.

Years down the line, when your child asks about their baby days, you'll have this photo journal to show them. It's a story told in pictures, a narrative of love, a keepsake that will warm your hearts.

Designing the Nursery Together

Designing the nursery is like setting the stage for a grand performance. It's about picking the right colors, choosing the perfect furniture, and creating a space that's warm, inviting, and ready to welcome the newest member of your family.

This activity is not just about aesthetics but also about teamwork. It's about making decisions together, compromising on choices, and building a space that reflects your shared dreams and hopes for your baby.

So, roll up your sleeves and dive into the world of nursery themes and crib choices. Let your creativity shine, let your love guide you, and together, create a haven for your little one.

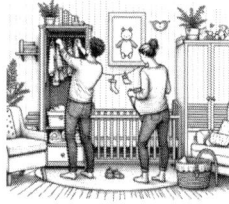

There you have it, future dad. A lineup of fun activities to bond with your unborn baby. These activities are not just for passing time or for creating Instagram-worthy posts. They're about forming a connection, about stepping into your role as a dad, and celebrating life's miracle. So, go ahead and have some fun. After all, pregnancy is not just about the destination but also about the joy of the journey.

Talking to Your Baby Bump: Why It Matters

Benefits of Talking to the Baby Bump

Alright, let's bust a myth right off the bat. The womb is not a soundproof booth. In fact, it's quite the opposite. Your unborn baby can hear sounds as early as the second trimester. So, when you're chatting away to the baby bump, your little one is all ears.

But it's not just about entertaining the baby with your dad jokes and shower singing sessions. Talking to the baby bump has some serious benefits. For starters, it's a fantastic way to bond with your baby. It's like a wireless connection, bridging the outside world with the coziness of the womb.

It also helps your baby recognize your voice. Studies have shown that newborns clearly prefer their mother's voice, but they're also pretty good at picking out their dad's dulcet tones. So, by talking to the baby bump, you're not just bonding with your baby but also giving them a head start in recognizing your voice.

What to Say to Your Baby Bump

Now, you might wonder, "What on earth do I say to a baby bump?" Well, the good news is your baby isn't critiquing your conversational skills. They're just soaking up the sound of your voice. So, you can pretty much say anything.

Share the highlights of your day, read a chapter from your favorite book, or tell them about the time you scored the winning goal in the high school soccer championship. The content doesn't matter; it's the sound of your voice, the rhythm of your speech, the melody of your tone that your baby is tuning into.

Best Times to Talk to Your Baby Bump

While there's no hard and fast rule about the best times to talk to the baby bump, it can be helpful to establish a routine. It could be a bedtime story ritual, a morning pep talk, or a post-dinner chat.

Having a routine not only creates a sense of familiarity for your baby but also helps you cultivate the habit of bonding with your baby. It's like setting a daily reminder to connect, bond, and build a relationship with your little one.

Encouraging Your Partner to Talk to the Baby Bump

And let's not forget about your partner. Encourage her to talk to the baby bump, too. After all, her voice is the one your baby hears the most. It's the familiar lullaby that lulls them to sleep, the soothing sound that calms them down.

Talking to the baby bump can also help your partner bond with the baby. It makes the pregnancy more real and more personal. It's not just about the baby growing inside her; it's about the bond growing between them.

So, future dad, get chatting. Break the ice with the baby bump, and share your stories, hopes, and dreams. And remember, each word, each sentence, each conversation is a thread, weaving a bond between you and your baby. A bond that starts in the womb and grows stronger with each passing day. A bond that's forged in love nurtured with care and strengthened with every "Hello, baby, it's Dad."

Keep in mind that you're not just talking to a baby bump. You're connecting with your child, rehearsing your role as a dad, preparing for the grand debut. So, go ahead and talk to the baby bump. Your voice is the first gift you give your child, the first expression of your love, the first note in the symphony of fatherhood.

The Magic of Feeling Baby Kicks

When to Expect Baby Kicks

Imagine waiting for the first snowflake of winter. The forecast says it's coming, but you don't know precisely when. That's what waiting for the first baby kicks feels like. The timeline can vary, but usually, your partner can start to feel the baby's movements as early as 18 weeks into the pregnancy. However, it might take a bit longer for first-time moms, potentially up until about week 22. These initial movements, often described as flutters or popcorn pops, are subtle, gentle, and easy to miss. But fear not, soon-to-be dad, these flutters will turn into unmistakable jabs and pokes as the weeks progress.

Interpreting Different Types of Movements

Now, let's decode the language of baby kicks. Just like Morse code, each kick, roll, or flutter carries a message. A series of quick, rhythmic movements might be your baby having a case of the hiccups. A sudden jab on the right side might be a playful kick or a punch. A rolling motion might be your baby changing position. And remember, just like adults, babies have their active and quiet periods. So, there will be times when your baby is having a dance party and times when they're taking a peaceful nap.

How to Encourage Baby Kicks

Alright, future dad, let's talk about how to get the party started. While you can't exactly control your baby's movements, there are a few tricks to encourage them to wiggle around. One way is for your partner to lay on her left side, increasing blood flow to the baby and stimulating movement. Having a cold drink or a small snack can also get the baby moving as they respond to changes in temperature and sugar levels.

Remember, these tricks are not about forcing movement but rather about creating an environment that encourages it. It's like playing your baby's favorite song to get them on the dance floor.

Sharing the Experience with Your Partner

Finally, let's talk about the most heartwarming part—sharing the experience with your partner. Feeling your baby move is one of the most magical experiences of pregnancy, and it's an experience you can share. So, the next time your partner feels a kick, ask her to place your hand on her belly. Feel the thump under your palm, the rhythm of movement, the miracle of life. It's a moment that connects all three of you, a moment of shared joy that you'll cherish forever.

And there you have it—a tour into the world of baby kicks. From understanding when to expect the first movements, decoding the types of movements, learning how to encourage kicks, to sharing the experience with your partner. It's a dance that unfolds over weeks, a rhythm that carries the heartbeat of your baby, a song that tells the story of life.

So, future dad, get ready to dance to this rhythm, to tune into this song, to celebrate the miracle of life. Because every kick, every roll, every flutter is a note in the symphony of your baby's growth, a beat in the rhythm of your journey to fatherhood.

And, as we close this chapter, remember the dance floor is now open, and your baby is ready to dance. So, step onto the dance floor, feel the rhythm, and let the magic of baby kicks sweep you off your feet. As we turn the page, we'll continue our dance into the world of understanding your partner's emotional changes. So, keep your dancing shoes on, future dad. The music is just getting started, and the best is yet to come.

Chapter 7:

Navigating the Foggy Path—Facing and Overcoming Fears as a First-Time Dad

Have you ever found yourself standing at the edge of a foggy path, uncertain about what lies ahead? That's a fitting description of how it feels to be a first-time dad. You're about to step into an unknown territory, filled with both excitement and anxiety. But remember, every dad, no matter how confident or experienced he seems now, has stood where you're standing. Let's take a moment to discuss some of the common fears you might be grappling with and remind you that you're not alone in this.

Common Fears of First-Time Dads: You're Not Alone

Fear of the Unknown

Remember the first time you rode a bike, drove a car, or started a new job? That butterfly-in-your-stomach feeling you had is what the fear of the unknown feels like. As a first-time dad, you're stepping onto a path you've never walked before. You're not sure what to expect, how you'll handle it, or what challenges lie ahead. It's like standing at the start of a maze, unsure of the twists and turns you'll encounter.

Fear of Not Being a Good Dad

Imagine you're at a karaoke night, and you've been handed the mic to sing a song you've never heard before. That's what fearing you won't be a good dad can feel like. You want to hit all the right notes, but you're not even sure what the tune is. It's a fear that stems from wanting the best for your child, wanting to guide them, protect them, and provide for them in the best way possible. Many first-time fathers grapple with the fear of not being a good dad, a concern that's widely recognized (American Psychological Association, n.d.).

Fear of Balancing Work and Family

Think of yourself as a juggler, trying to keep multiple balls in the air. One ball is your work, another is your family, and yet another is your personal time. The fear of balancing work and family is like worrying about keeping all those balls in the air without dropping any. It's about wondering how you'll fulfill your professional responsibilities while being a present, active father at home.

Fear of Financial Pressure

Picture yourself standing in front of a slot machine, watching the numbers spin, hoping for a jackpot. That's what the fear of financial pressure can feel like. You're about to take on the financial responsibility of another human being. The costs can seem overwhelming, from diapers and baby gear to future college funds. It's like staring at a long grocery receipt, wondering how a tiny human can need so many things.

So, there you have it, soon-to-be dad. These fears you're feeling? They're more common than you think. They don't make you weak or unprepared. They make you human. They show that you care, that you want to do well, that you're invested in this new role you're about to take on. So, take a deep breath, square your shoulders, and let's move forward. Because guess what? You've got this. You're stronger than you think, braver than you believe, and more prepared than you feel.

And this foggy path you're standing on? It leads to a beautiful destination. So, let's take that first step together.

Financial Planning

Planning for the baby's grand entrance is like navigating a financial rollercoaster, but fear not—I've got the lowdown!

First off, let's dissect your moolah situation. List your cash sources and monthly spending—get down to the nitty-gritty. Then, beef up or start that emergency fund. Think of it as a superhero cape for your wallet in case life throws you a curveball.

Now, health insurance. Brace yourself for deductibles, co-pays, and all those fancy terms. It's like learning a secret language, but crack the code, and you'll be ready for the medical maze.

Future expenses: think education, soccer classes, maybe even a mini rock climbing adventure. It's like forecasting your financial weather—grab an umbrella for those unexpected downpours.

Insurance check! Life insurance is your family's superhero cape. Update beneficiaries like you're handing out VIP passes to a secret party.

Estate planning: create a will, designate guardianship, and add a dash of drama. Just kidding, keep it simple. And throw in a healthcare proxy for good measure.

Childcare costs are like a sneak attack. Daycare, nanny, or grandma—estimate the damage and prepare for a friendly budget battle.

Finally, review and adjust. Parenthood is like an improv show—be ready to roll with the punches. Regular money check-ins with your partner keep the laughs coming and the financial ship steady. Remember, this financial rodeo is a team effort. So, saddle up, partner, and let the baby budgeting bonanza begin!

Saving Tips

Let's talk about making money moves for the baby on the way—it's easier than you think! First up, create a special savings spot just for baby stuff, like a superhero lair for your cash. Break down what you need to save for, set goals, and suddenly, saving becomes a fun game. Check out your budget and find some extra cash by trimming here and there—think of it as a budget superhero saving the day, one dollar at a time. Essentials first, like a safe crib and diapers, and then you can sprinkle in the cute baby outfits. Hunt for deals, try second-hand options and make a baby registry if you have a shower. It's like getting the baby gear you need without the guesswork. Look into government programs for extra help, and if you're up for it, try a side hustle for more baby fund cash. Cook at home, cancel unused subscriptions, and set up automatic savings like a money ninja. And don't forget, if unpaid parental leave is on the horizon, start saving early. With these tricks, you'll be a baby-saving pro without breaking a sweat.

Strategies to Manage Parenting Anxieties

Practicing Mindfulness

In the hustle and bustle of preparing for a baby, it's easy to get caught up in a storm of worries and what-ifs. To help reel in these anxieties, consider the concept of mindfulness. It's like taking a magnifying glass to the present moment and examining it with curiosity and without judgment.

Mindfulness practices can help mitigate parental anxieties (Headspace, n.d.). Mindfulness allows you to acknowledge your anxieties without letting them take the driver's seat. It's like watching clouds drift across the sky, observing their shapes and patterns, but not getting swept up in the wind.

There are many ways to incorporate mindfulness into your daily routine. You could start your day with five minutes of mindful breathing, focusing on the sensation of the breath entering and leaving your body. Or you could practice mindful eating, savoring each bite of your meal. It's about finding pockets of peace amid the chaos, grounding yourself in the here and now.

Seeking Support From Other Dads

There's a certain comfort in shared experiences. That's why reaching out to other dads—especially those who've recently had babies—can be a game-changer. Their fresh insights and firsthand knowledge can shed light on your own anxieties, and their reassurances can help put your worries into perspective. Seeking support from other dads who have recently experienced fatherhood can provide reassurance and practical tips (Fatherly, n.d.).

Think of it as swapping notes with teammates. They can share their winning strategies, their rookie mistakes, and their unexpected discoveries. This camaraderie can ease your anxieties and help you feel more prepared for your new role.

You could join a local dads' group, participate in online forums, or simply chat with friends who are fathers. Remember, every dad's experience is unique, but there are common threads that weave through all of their stories.

Regular Exercise

Exercise is a proven stress-buster, and it can play a crucial role in managing your parenting anxieties. Regular physical exercise is beneficial in managing stress and anxiety for expectant fathers (Healthline, n.d.). It's like breaking the anxiety chain with a surge of endorphins, those feel-good chemicals that boost your mood and clear your mind.

You could go for a run, hit the gym, shoot some hoops, or even shake a leg to your favorite tunes in your living room. The type of exercise isn't as important as the regularity. It's about moving your body, breaking a sweat, and shaking off the stress.

As an added bonus, regular exercise can help you stay fit and healthy, which will come in handy when you're chasing after your little one in a couple of years!

Open Communication With Your Partner

Last but not least, don't underestimate the power of open communication with your partner. You're both in this together, after all. Sharing your anxieties can help lighten your emotional load, and listening to your partner's concerns can provide you with a fresh perspective.

It's like holding up a mirror to your worries and viewing them from a different angle. What seemed like a mountain might turn out to be a molehill, and what you assumed was a solo concern could be a shared worry.

Set aside quiet moments for these heart-to-heart chats. Speak honestly, listen empathetically, and remember that it's okay to be vulnerable. These conversations can not only ease your anxieties but also strengthen your bond as you prepare to welcome your baby into the world.

There you have it—a toolbox of strategies to manage your parenting anxieties. From practicing mindfulness to seeking support from other dads, exercising regularly, and communicating openly with your partner, each tool offers a unique way to navigate your worries. They're not magic wands that will make your anxieties disappear, but they can help you manage them, understand them, and maybe even learn from them. So, go ahead and give them a try. After all, becoming a dad is not just about bringing a baby into the world; it's also about growing, evolving, and learning along the way.

How to Cultivate a Positive Mindset

Daily Affirmations

Picture yourself standing in front of a mirror, looking into your own eyes, and repeating powerful, positive statements to yourself. Sounds simple, doesn't it? Yet this practice, known as daily affirmations, can be a game-changer in cultivating a positive mindset.

Affirmations are like pep talks you give yourself, a way of programming your mind to believe in your capabilities and strengths. Daily affirmations can positively impact mental health and well-being (PositivePsychology.com, n.d.). As a future dad, your affirmations could be statements like "I am prepared to be a great dad," "I am capable of balancing work and family," or "I am ready to embrace the changes ahead."

These aren't just empty words you're parroting. They're powerful declarations that can help you replace negative thoughts with positive ones, shift your mindset, and boost your confidence. So, make a habit of starting your day with a few affirmations. Because when you change your thoughts, you change your world.

Visualization Techniques

Close your eyes and imagine holding your baby for the first time. The softness of their skin, the warmth of their body, the rhythm of their breath. This practice of creating a mental image is called visualization, and it's a powerful technique to cultivate a positive mindset.

Visualization is like a rehearsal in your mind, an opportunity to experience and familiarize yourself with future events. As a soon-to-be dad, you can visualize various scenarios—from changing diapers and soothing a crying baby to playing with your toddler in the park.

By visualizing these scenarios, you're not just preparing yourself for fatherhood but also creating positive anticipation for the experiences to come. So, take a few minutes each day to visualize, rehearse, and connect with your future self.

Celebrating Small Wins

Remember when you scored your first goal in a soccer game or aced a difficult test? That rush of joy you felt is the power of celebrating small wins. As you prepare for fatherhood, there will be numerous small wins along the way, and each is worth celebrating.

Did you manage to put together the crib without losing a single screw? Well, that's a win right there. Survive your inaugural prenatal class without hitting the floor? Bingo, another win. And, hey, if you've finally cracked the code on onesies versus rompers, consider that a victory dance-worthy moment.

Celebrating these small wins isn't about throwing yourself a party for every little thing. It's about acknowledging your progress, no matter how tiny, and letting it be the fuel for your confidence and positivity. So, don't hold out for the grand, applause-worthy moments to break out the metaphorical confetti.

Picture this journey into fatherhood as a series of victories, each one adding a star to your dad cape. Whether it's mastering the art of diaper changing or successfully assembling baby gear, these accomplishments are your superhero badges. And guess what? They're just as important as the big, spotlight-stealing feats.

So, revel in these small victories, embrace the learning curve, and let each win be a reminder that you're acing this dad thing, one triumph at a time. In the end, it's the collection of these small wins that paint the vibrant canvas of your fatherhood journey. Celebrate every step, every milestone, every win on your path to fatherhood.

Embracing the Journey of Fatherhood

Think back to a difficult task you took on. Maybe it was running a marathon or learning a new language. It was hard, perhaps even overwhelming at times. But you didn't just focus on the finish line; you embraced the entire process, the highs, the lows, and everything in between.

The same goes for the journey of fatherhood. It's not just about holding your baby at the finish line; it's about embracing the entire process, from the pregnancy and birth to the sleepless nights and first steps.

Embracing the journey means accepting that there will be challenges but also knowing that the joy and love you'll experience will far outweigh them. It's about seeing every stumble as an opportunity to learn and every challenge as a chance to grow.

So, as you stand on the threshold of fatherhood, take a deep breath and embrace the journey. You're not just becoming a dad; you're also evolving as a person, and that's something to look forward to.

The Power of a Support System: Don't Be Afraid to Seek Help

Building a Network of Support

Imagine you're about to build a house. Now, would you even think about tackling such a monumental task all on your own? Probably not. You'd gather a dream team—architects, contractors, and plumbers—experts in their respective fields. The same principle applies to your parenting journey. Getting a strong support crew is like hiring your team, ready to help you set the foundation for your new role as a dad.

A strong support system, including healthcare professionals, mental health counselors, and parenting experts, is vital for new fathers

(American Academy of Pediatrics, n.d.). They're the go-to people for professional advice, the ones who can give you reliable answers when you're scratching your head with questions.

First up, healthcare professionals are like the architects of your parenting plan. They know the ins and outs of keeping your partner and soon-to-arrive little one healthy. From checkups to post-baby care, they've got the know-how to guide you.

Then, there are mental health counselors—your emotional helpers. Parenting brings all sorts of feelings, and having someone who knows the ropes can make a big difference. They help you strengthen your emotional base so you can handle the ups and downs like a pro.

Don't forget the lactation consultants and your feeding system experts. Feeding your new baby is super important, and these consultants are like the fix-it crew, ready to solve any feeding hiccups. Whether it's breastfeeding or bottle-feeding, they keep things running smoothly.

Last but not least, the parenting pros—your overall project managers. They're the ones who know everything about baby sleep, soothing techniques, and more. Whenever you're puzzled about baby stuff, they're the ones with the tips and tricks.

Building this support crew isn't just about making life easier; it's a smart move. These folks aren't just there for the big moments; they're the ones you can turn to for all the little details. They're like your experts on baby-proofing or figuring out the diaper game.

So, think of creating your support crew as a necessary move, not just a nice-to-have. It's like saying, "Hey, I'm ready for this dad thing, and I'm going to get all the help I need." It's not admitting defeat; it's showing you're committed to being the awesome dad you want to be. So, go on, reach out, and build your own support crew. It's not a sign of weakness; it's a smart way to make sure your dad journey stands on the shoulders of wisdom and experience.

Joining a New Dads Group

Recall the last time you became part of a club or a team. There's that unique feeling of camaraderie, the shared journey, the comfort of belonging. Now, think about joining a group specifically for new dads—it's like entering a club where everyone is embarking on the exhilarating and somewhat nerve-wracking adventure of first-time fatherhood.

These new dads groups act as a haven, a space where you can openly share your fears, uncertainties, and victories. It's a treasure trove of practical tips, emotional support, and ingenious dad hacks. Joining new dads' groups can offer peer support and reduce feelings of isolation (The Bump, n.d.). Imagine having a crew of fellow dads who understand exactly what you're going through, offering insights and encouragement along the way.

Being part of such a group provides a safety net for expressing the thoughts that might be swirling in your mind. Whether it's the worry about changing diapers or the excitement of witnessing your baby's first steps, these dads have likely been there, done that, and can offer guidance.

Moreover, these groups serve as a platform to cultivate friendships with dads who are in the same boat as you. It's an opportunity to build connections with those who are experiencing the unique blend of joy and chaos that comes with being a new dad. These connections might just lead to future playdates for your little ones, creating a network of support not just for you but also for your kids as they grow.

So, think of joining a new dads group as more than just a social activity. It's a dynamic space where you share the highs and lows of fatherhood, gather valuable advice, and form lasting connections. It's your personalized club for navigating the uncharted waters of parenthood, ensuring you're not alone in this exciting, daunting, and wonderful journey.

Leaning on Friends and Family

Think back to those carefree days of childhood when your best friend was the go-to person for tackling tricky math problems or soothing a scraped knee. Well, it's time to tap into that support system again, but this time, with your friends and family. They're your personal cheerleaders, sounding boards, and helping hands—your ultimate support crew.

When the parenting journey gets a bit overwhelming, don't be shy about reaching out for assistance. Whether it's for a bit of babysitting relief, a hand in meal prep, or simply a good old venting session over a cup of coffee, your friends and family are there to lend a helping hand. Just as it took a village to raise a child in traditional wisdom, your friends and family play crucial roles in your modern-day village. Friends and family play a crucial role in providing emotional and practical support (National Institutes of Health, n.d.).

Consider them your backup squad, ready to step in when you need a breather or a friendly ear. Parenting is no solo act, and acknowledging that you might need a bit of help is a strength, not a weakness. These are the people who've seen you through thick and thin, and now, they're ready to join you in this new chapter of parenthood.

So, don't forget to lean on your friends and family, just like you did in those carefree days. They're not just your support system; they're an integral part of the village that contributes to the growth and well-being of your child. Whether it's sharing the load or celebrating the wins, your village is there to make the parenting journey a bit lighter, a bit more enjoyable, and a whole lot more memorable. After all, raising a child is not just about the parents—it's a team effort, and your friends and family are your invaluable teammates.

Seeking Professional Help if Needed

Finally, let's talk about a crucial piece of the puzzle—professional help. Sometimes, despite your best efforts, you might find yourself struggling with feelings of overwhelm, anxiety, or depression. Seeking professional help is important if you're struggling with overwhelming emotions (Mental Health America, n.d.). Think of it as calling in the reinforcements when things get tough.

This might involve engaging in conversations with a mental health professional, participating in a support group, or consulting your healthcare provider for guidance. There's no shame in reaching out. In fact, it's a sign of strength and shows your commitment to being the best dad you can be.

To wrap things up, this is the blueprint for building your support system. Remember, becoming a dad isn't a solo expedition. It's a team sport, and you've got a whole squad ready to back you up. So, reach out, connect, and remember—you're not alone in this. You're part of a community, a network, a family. And together, you're building more than just a network of support. You're building a home filled with love, care, and shared joy.

With every page and chapter, you're learning, growing, and preparing to be the best dad you can be. So, keep reading, keep learning, and keep growing.

Chapter 8:

The Domestic Dojo—Preparing Your Home for the Little One

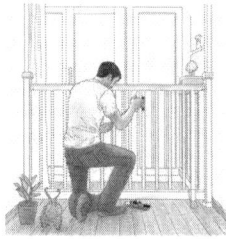

Imagine you've just been handed the keys to an ancient castle. It's grand, it's beautiful, and it's yours to protect. Now, replace that castle with your home, and consider the upcoming arrival of your baby as the precious treasure you're safeguarding. Your mission, should you choose to accept it (and let's face it, you don't really have a choice), is to transform your home into a domestic dojo—a haven that's safe, secure, and ready for its newest occupant. Grab your safety gear, future dad, and let's get to work!

How to Baby-Proof Your Home: A Practical Guide

The martial art of baby-proofing is not taught in any dojo, but fear not because this guide has got you covered. And remember, baby-proofing is less about achieving aesthetic perfection and more about ensuring practical safety (CPSC, n.d.; Cleveland Clinic, 2023; National Safety Council, n.d.).

Securing Furniture and TVs

Picture this: You're a secret agent, and your mission is to prevent a potential "furniture avalanche." Your targets? Any piece of furniture or appliance that could potentially tip over, such as bookcases, dressers, and TVs. The tool for your mission? Furniture straps and brackets.

Install these safety devices to secure top-heavy furniture and TVs to the wall. It's like roping down a wild stallion, keeping it from causing havoc. Remember, the lower shelves of bookcases can be very tempting for a curious crawler, so keep them free of small objects that could be a choking hazard.

Installing Baby Gates

Next in your arsenal of baby-proofing techniques is the installation of baby gates. Think of them as mini drawbridges in your domestic castle, keeping your adventurous knight or maiden from venturing into potentially dangerous territories (CPSC, n.d.).

Install baby gates at the top and bottom of any staircases and in the doorways of rooms with hazards. It's like setting up checkpoints in a video game, controlling where your little one can venture. And remember, secure mounting is key when it comes to baby gates. A pressure-mounted gate might work fine for doorways, but for top-of-stair use, nothing beats the security of a hardware-mounted gate.

Locking Cabinets and Drawers

Now, let's tackle those sneaky little hazards known as cabinets and drawers. To a baby, they're like hidden treasure chests begging to be explored. Your job? To keep those treasures under lock and key.

Place safety latches on cabinets and drawers, especially those within your baby's reach. Pay special attention to those storing cleaning supplies, medication, or sharp utensils. It's like setting up a security system for the crown jewels, except in this case, the jewels are everyday household items that pose risks to your baby.

Covering Electrical Outlets

Last but not least, turn your attention to those tantalizing little holes in the wall—electrical outlets. To your baby, they're like mysterious caves just waiting to be probed by tiny fingers or metal objects (Cleveland Clinic, 2023).

Invest in outlet covers or safety plugs to keep these potential hazards out of reach. It's like putting up a "No Entry" sign on a dangerous path, guiding your little explorer away from harm.

To sum it up, future dad, a step-by-step guide to transforming your home into a domestic dojo—a safe haven for your little one to grow, explore, and conquer milestones (not furniture). So, roll up your sleeves, summon your inner handyman, and let the baby-proofing begin!

Assembling Baby Furniture: A Fun DIY Project

Choosing the Right Furniture

Alright, future dad, imagine you're back in your childhood, standing in a toy store and eyeing the coolest new playset. Now, fast forward to the present; replace the toy store with a baby store and the playset with baby furniture. It's time to choose your baby's first bed, wardrobe, and changing station.

When choosing baby furniture, keep in mind the three S's—safety, size, and style. Safety is paramount—look for furniture with no sharp edges and ensure it adheres to safety standards. Size is crucial, too—you want to choose furniture that fits well in your nursery without making it feel cramped. Finally, style—choose furniture that compliments your nursery's decor, creating a warm, welcoming environment.

Safety Tips for Assembling Furniture

Now, it's time to put on your DIY hat. Assembling furniture can be a fun project, but it's also one that requires careful attention to safety. So, here are a few tips to keep in mind.

Firstly, follow the instructions. They might seem like a boring read, but they're your roadmap to a safe and sturdy assembly. Secondly, use the right tools. Trying to use a butter knife as a screwdriver might seem like a creative solution, but it won't result in a sturdy piece of furniture. Lastly, double-check your work. Once assembled, give the furniture a good shake to ensure it's secure and stable.

Making it a Team Effort

Remember those school projects where you and your buddies would team up to build the best model volcano? Well, assembling baby furniture can be a team effort, too.

Invite your partner to join in. She can read out the instructions while you do the heavy lifting or vice versa. Working together not only makes the process quicker and more enjoyable but also creates shared memories. It's like you're both artists collaborating on a masterpiece for your little one.

Adding Personal Touches

Finally, it's time to add some personal touches. This is where you can let your creativity shine.

Perhaps you could paint the dresser in a shade that matches the nursery or add some cute decals to the wardrobe. Maybe you want to hang a mobile over the crib or place a soft, cuddly teddy bear on the changing table. These personal touches are like the cherry on top of the sundae, adding a dash of love and personality to the furniture.

So, here it is, soon-to-be dad. You've chosen the right furniture, followed safety guidelines during assembly, made it a team effort, and added personal touches. Your domestic dojo is now one step closer to being ready for its newest member. So, take a moment to admire your handiwork. You're not just assembling furniture; you're building a cozy, welcoming world for your little one. And that's something to be proud of.

The Essential New Dad Checklist: Your Trusty Guide

Baby Gear Must-Haves

Setting sail on the sea of fatherhood requires a well-packed ship. The first item on your checklist? Baby gear.

- **car seat**: Non-negotiable and needed right from the start. Ensure it's government-approved and installed correctly.

- **stroller**: For those leisurely walks or quick trips to the store, a sturdy and easy-to-navigate stroller is a worthy investment.

  A pro-tip for you: Consider the Doona brand stroller/car seat. It's a nifty combo of both! This gem serves as a car seat, and the magic happens when you pull it out of the car—the wheels swing right from underneath, instantly turning it into a stroller.

- **baby carrier**: For those times your little one wants to snuggle close while you have tasks to accomplish, a baby carrier is a lifesaver. My personal preference is the Ergobaby Omni 360 brand. It stands out for its SoftFlex Mesh, ensuring optimal airflow to keep both you and your baby cool and dry throughout the day. What I love is that it adapts as your baby grows from newborn to toddler. It's incredibly versatile, allowing you to position it from any angle effortlessly. You can choose to carry your baby outward or inward from the front, switch to a backpack style, or even use it as a hip seat at your side.

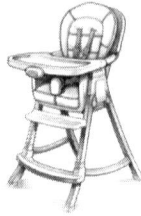

- **crib and mattress**: Your baby's slumber spot needs to be safe, snug, and up to code with current safety standards.

- **high chair**: Not immediately necessary, but around the six-month mark, you'll be glad to have it.

- **baby monitor**: For peace of mind during nap time and beyond.

Setting Up the Nursery

Next on your checklist is creating a peaceful sanctuary for your baby.

- **choose a theme**: Whether you're all about the animals or fixated on flowers, picking a theme can streamline design decisions.

- **paint**: Opt for a nursery-friendly paint—preferably one that's easy to clean and free of harmful chemicals.

- **functional furniture**: Apart from the crib, consider a comfy chair (for those late-night feeds), a changing table, and storage for clothes and toys.

- **lighting**: Soft, calming lights can make bedtime routines a whole lot easier.

- **decorations**: Here's where you can let your theme shine. Wall decals, mobiles, curtains—the sky's the limit!

Stocking Up on Diapers and Wipes

Diapers and wipes will become your new best friends, so stock up!

- **diapers**: Whether you opt for cloth or disposable, having a stash of diapers at hand is essential. For a newborn, aim for 10-12 diapers a day.

- **wipes**: Perfect for diaper changes, messy meals, and general clean-ups.

Certain states have diaper banks that offer a supply of diapers, usually enough to last for a few weeks. While there might be a lengthy line to acquire these diapers and wipes, it's worthwhile if you have the time, and it contributes to building up your stockpile. Check with your local resources to find out what services are available in your area.

Planning for Paternity Leave

Taking time off work when your baby arrives gives you precious bonding time and helps you support your partner.

- **know your rights**: Look into your company's policies and the laws in your country to understand your entitlements.

- **plan ahead**: Discuss your paternity leave plans with your employer well in advance of your baby's due date.

- **set boundaries**: If possible, limit work calls and emails during your leave to fully concentrate on your family.

Scheduling Pediatrician Appointments

Your baby's first doctor's visit typically happens in the first week after birth.

- **find a pediatrician**: Before your baby arrives, research and select a pediatrician. Consider factors like location, office hours, and approach to healthcare.

- **schedule the first visit**: Typically occurring three to five days after birth. If you don't have a pediatrician yet, rest assured that your baby will be seen by one at the hospital. Some parents prefer sticking to the same pediatrician for continuity, ensuring the doctor has a comprehensive history of your baby from day one. Don't worry if you haven't chosen one beforehand. Before the visit, it's helpful to jot down any questions or concerns you may have.

And there you have it—your go-to checklist as a soon-to-be dad. Each tick on this list brings you one step closer to being fully prepped for your new addition, from baby gear to doctor visits. Remember, preparation is not just about the items you gather or the tasks you complete. It's about the love and care behind each action, the eager anticipation of meeting your little one, and the growing confidence in your abilities as a dad. So, keep ticking off those tasks, knowing that with each checkmark, you're not just preparing for your baby's arrival; you're also embracing your role as a dad.

What to Pack for the Hospital Bag: The Ultimate Guide

Essentials for Mom

You've heard the old saying, "Mother knows best." But when it comes to packing for the hospital, even the most prepared mom-to-be can overlook a few things. It's worth noting that many hospitals have these items readily available, but it's a smart move to bring your own, just in case. Plus, having your preferred brands for the things you like is an extra touch of comfort.

- **clothing**: Comfort is key. Pack a lightweight robe, a few pairs of non-skid socks, nursing bras, and nipple balm if you are planning to breastfeed. Don't forget a going-home outfit— something loose and comfy will do the trick.

- **toiletries**: Travel-size shampoo, conditioner, body wash, toothpaste, and a toothbrush are must-haves. Add in a lip balm and unscented lotion to combat hospital air dryness.

- **comfort items**: Consider packing a favorite pillow or blanket to make the hospital environment feel a bit more like home.

Essentials for Baby

Alright, future dad, it's time to pack some pint-sized essentials for your little one's grand entrance into the world.

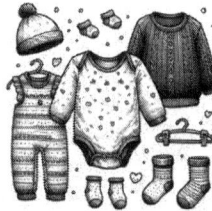

- **clothing**: Pack a couple of onesies, sleepers, and swaddling blankets. Don't forget the adorable going-home outfit and a weather-appropriate cover if needed.

- **diapers and wipes**: While most hospitals provide these, it doesn't hurt to have a few of your own on hand.

- **car seat**: Technically, it is not in the bag, but it is absolutely crucial for the ride home. Make sure it's properly installed ahead of time.

Essentials for Dad

While this might feel like an adventure in a foreign land for you, future dad, packing a few essentials can make the hospital stay more comfortable.

- **clothing**: Pack a change of clothes. Hospitals aren't known for their five-star sleeping arrangements, so comfy pajamas are a must.

- **snacks and drinks**: Hospital food isn't exactly gourmet. Pack some of your favorite snacks and drinks to keep your energy up. Additionally, toss in some coins for the vending machine. It's a small detail, but having a snack readily available can be a lifesaver during those late-night cravings or moments of hunger between meals.

- **entertainment**: There might be a lot of waiting around. A book, tablet, or laptop can help pass the time.

- **phone charger**: Since numerous family members will likely want updates on both mom and the baby, keeping your phone charged is crucial. Not only will this ensure that you don't miss any incoming calls, but it's also essential for capturing precious moments by taking pictures and videos of your little bundle of joy. So, having a charged phone becomes a dual necessity, allowing you to stay connected with loved ones and capture the delightful memories of your newborn.

Remember, while the hospital may provide some necessities, having your own comfort items and essentials on hand can make the experience more familiar and tailored to your preferences.

Important Documents to Bring

No mission is complete without the right paperwork.

- **ID and insurance information**: Don't forget your driver's license, insurance card, and a copy of your birth plan if you have one.

- **pediatrician's contact information**: The hospital will ask for this information so they can send over records of your baby's birth.

Alright, future dad, you're all set! You've got your baby-proofed home, your hospital bag is packed, and you're ready to welcome your little one into the world. Just remember, while the preparation is important, the most crucial thing you're bringing to the hospital isn't in your bag; it's the love and excitement in your heart. So, as you step into this new chapter of life, know that you're ready, you're prepared, and you're about to embark on the greatest adventure of all—becoming a dad.

Up ahead, we'll explore the postpartum period—a transformative time that brings its own set of adventures and challenges. But with the preparation you've already done, you're more than ready to face whatever comes your way. So, onward, we go into the captivating world of life after birth.

Chapter 9:

The Postpartum Puzzle—Putting Together the Pieces

Picture a jigsaw puzzle. It starts with hundreds of scattered pieces, each unique, each holding a fragment of the bigger picture. Slowly, you start connecting the pieces, recognizing patterns, and discovering connections. Postpartum recovery is a bit like that jigsaw puzzle. It's about navigating physical changes, hormonal shifts, and emotional transformations—all different pieces of the same puzzle.

As a soon-to-be dad, it's crucial to understand these postpartum changes. Not only will this knowledge help you support your partner, but it will also equip you to adapt to your new role as a dad. So, let's roll up our sleeves and start assembling this postpartum puzzle, piece by piece.

Understanding Postpartum Recovery: The Physical Aspects

Healing After Childbirth

Childbirth, whether vaginal or via C-section, is a significant physical event. Like an athlete, your partner's body needs time to recover and heal after a strenuous game.

After a vaginal delivery, discomfort in the perineal area (the region between the vagina and rectum) is common. Your partner may also experience contractions, often referred to as afterpains, as her uterus shrinks back to its pre-pregnancy size. These afterpains can feel like mild to intense cramping and usually last a few days *(The Mother Baby Center, n.d.)*.

In the case of a C-section, your partner will be recovering from major abdominal surgery. This involves healing of the incision, management of postoperative pain, and gradual return to normal activities. It's crucial to remember that recovery timelines vary for every woman, and patience is key *(APTA Pelvic Health, 2023)*.

Hormonal Changes Post-Delivery

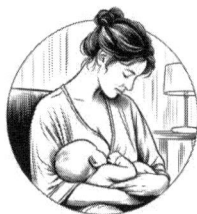

Just like a rollercoaster ride, your partner's hormones take a steep plunge right after delivery. Levels of estrogen and progesterone, the hormones that maintain pregnancy, drop dramatically. At the same time, levels of other hormones like prolactin and oxytocin rise to facilitate breastfeeding and mother-baby bonding.

This hormonal flip can have various physical effects. Your partner may experience night sweats or hot flashes as her body adjusts to the hormonal changes. She may also notice changes in her skin and hair due to these fluctuating hormone levels.

Postpartum Body Changes

Imagine your body morphing over nine months and then having to morph back in a much shorter time. That's what postpartum body changes are like.

Your partner's body will gradually change as it recovers from pregnancy and childbirth. She may notice changes in her breasts, particularly if she's breastfeeding. Her belly will slowly shrink, although it might take time for her to return to her pre-pregnancy shape. She may also experience changes in her menstrual cycle when it resumes.

Remember, these changes are part of the normal postpartum recovery process. They represent the remarkable resilience and adaptability of the female body. Encourage your partner to embrace these changes and to be patient with her body as it heals and adjusts.

Remember to be patient, supportive, and understanding as you're piecing together the postpartum puzzle. Your partner's body has undergone an incredible transformation to bring your baby into the world. Understanding these changes and providing empathetic support will help her navigate this postpartum period with confidence and ease. As you assemble each piece of the puzzle, you're not just understanding postpartum recovery; you're also stepping into your role as a supportive partner and a caring dad. And that's a picture worth piecing together.

The Emotional Roller Coaster: Postpartum Mood Changes

Understanding Postpartum Depression

Imagine a cloud-filled sky on a day when the weather forecast promised sunshine. That's somewhat akin to what postpartum depression (PPD) feels like. It's an unexpected visitor, often arriving a few weeks after childbirth, casting a shadow over what should be a joyous time (Mayo Clinic, n.d.).

PPD is more than just the "baby blues," which is a milder, shorter-lived emotional reaction experienced by many new mothers. It's a serious mood disorder that involves feelings of extreme sadness, anxiety, and fatigue. It can make it difficult for new mothers to perform daily care activities or form a loving bond with their baby (Allina Health, n.d.; Johns Hopkins Medicine, n.d.).

In some cases, postpartum depression may resolve within a few weeks or months, especially with appropriate treatment, which may include therapy, support groups, medication, or a combination of these. However, for others, postpartum depression may persist for a more extended period, and without intervention, it may become chronic.

It's important to remember that PPD is not a sign of weakness or a character flaw. It doesn't mean your partner is unfit or unloving as a mother. It's a medical condition that requires treatment, just like any physical ailment.

New dads, here's a heads up: it's common for most moms not to readily admit if they're dealing with postpartum depression. This might make it a bit challenging to recognize, so it's crucial to be attentive and supportive during this period. If you notice any signs or concerns, approaching the topic with care and openness can encourage her to share what she's going through and seek the help she may need.

Recognizing Signs of Postpartum Anxiety

Consider a smoke alarm that keeps going off despite no sign of fire. That's somewhat similar to what postpartum anxiety (PPA) feels like. It's a constant state of worry, fear, or unease that disrupts daily life—a false alarm that refuses to turn off.

PPA can manifest in various ways. Your partner might constantly worry about the baby's health or safety, or she could be plagued by disturbing thoughts she can't shake off. She may also experience physical symptoms like a racing heart, hot flashes, or dizziness.

Keep an eye out for signs of PPA. It often goes unrecognized because some level of anxiety is expected for new parents. However, if your partner's worries are constant, excessive, or interfere with her ability to care for the baby or herself, it's time to seek help.

Postpartum Mood Swings and Their Impact

Picture a pendulum swinging back and forth. At one end is elation, and at the other, despair. That's a bit of what postpartum mood swings can feel like. One moment, your partner might be overjoyed, gazing adoringly at your baby, and the next, she could be in tears, overwhelmed by the enormity of parenthood.

These mood swings are largely due to hormonal changes after childbirth. As her hormone levels fluctuate, so do her emotions. It's like being on a seesaw that refuses to stay still.

Mood swings can make the postpartum period feel like an emotional minefield. Your partner may feel like she's losing control, which can be quite distressing. Providing emotional support during this time is crucial. Let her know that it's okay to feel this way and that these mood swings are a normal part of the postpartum period.

In conclusion, the postpartum period can be an emotional roller coaster ride. Understanding the signs of PPD and PPA, as well as navigating mood swings, is crucial to supporting your partner during this time. Remember, these conditions do not reflect your partner's ability to be a good mother. They are medical conditions that require care and treatment. So, be patient, be supportive, and most importantly, let her know she's not alone. With time, treatment, and a whole lot of love, the clouds will clear, revealing the sunshine that's been there all along.

A Compassionate Companion: Supporting Your Partner's Postpartum Recovery

Providing Emotional Support

Let's circle back to an earlier analogy—the emotional roller coaster. As your partner rides the ups and downs of postpartum emotions, she's going to need a steadfast companion. That's where you, future dad, step in. Your role is to be the steady hand that guides her through the loop-the-loops, the reassuring voice that calms her during the steep drops, and the constant presence that celebrates the exhilarating highs with her.

Talk to her about her feelings, create a safe space for her to express her emotions freely, and validate her experiences. A simple "I'm here for you," "You're doing great," or "It's okay to feel this way" can go a long way in making her feel supported. Remember, emotional support isn't about fixing things or finding solutions; it's about listening, empathizing, and standing by her side no matter what.

Assisting With Baby Care

Now, let's turn our attention to the bundle of joy that's just arrived. Babies, while adorable, can be quite a handful. They require round-the-clock care, and for a recovering mom, managing it all can be overwhelming. This is where your dad abilities come into play.

Take charge of diaper changes, bottle feedings, and soothing sessions. Become a master swaddler, a pro at burping the baby, and an expert at deciphering different types of cries. Share the night shifts so your partner gets a chance to rest. It's not just about easing her load; it's also a fantastic way for you to bond with your baby and actively participate in their care.

Encouraging Rest and Self-Care

Picture a car running on empty, trying to navigate a steep hill. It sputters, it struggles, and eventually, it stops. That's what happens when we neglect rest and self-care—we run out of fuel. Postpartum recovery requires ample rest, and as the supportive partner, you need to ensure your better half gets plenty of it.

Encourage her to sleep when the baby sleeps, even if it's midday. Take over baby care duties so she can have a relaxing bath or read a book. Remind her to eat nutritious meals and stay hydrated. Small gestures like making her a cup of tea, giving her a shoulder massage, or simply holding the baby so she can have a break can make a world of difference.

In the turbulence of new parenthood, self-care often takes a back seat. But remember, a well-rested, well-cared-for mom is better equipped to care for the baby. So, make rest and self-care non-negotiable elements of your partner's postpartum recovery. Because, as they say, you can't pour from an empty cup.

As you navigate the path of postpartum recovery with your partner, remember that patience, understanding, and empathy are your trusty guides. Every woman's recovery journey is unique, and there's no set timeline or roadmap to follow. Your role is to walk beside her, offering your unwavering support, celebrating her progress, and reminding her of the incredible strength she possesses. After all, she's not just recovering from childbirth; she's also stepping into her new role as a mom. And just like you, she's learning, growing, and discovering her strengths. So, hold her hand, have her back, and together, navigate the postpartum path—not as two individuals, but as a team.

As we transition to the next chapter, keep in mind that you're not merely a spectator in this postpartum journey; you're actively engaged. Every action matters from providing emotional support and assisting with baby care to encouraging rest and self-care. Each diaper changed, each comforting word, and each freshly brewed cup of tea is a testament to your love and dedication. So, keep going, future dad. With every step, every action, and each passing day, you're not just supporting your partner's recovery; you're also embracing your role as a dad. It's a journey worth cherishing.

The Importance of Patience and Understanding

Exhibiting Empathy Amidst Recovery

Picture this: It's a cold winter's day, and you're offering your partner a warm blanket, a steaming cup of cocoa, and a comforting hug. That's what showing empathy during postpartum recovery feels like. It's about offering warmth and understanding during a time that can often feel cold and confusing.

Your partner is not just recovering from childbirth; she's also navigating the emotional labyrinth of becoming a mom. She's adjusting to sleepless nights, frequent feedings, and the constant needs of a newborn. She's dealing with hormonal fluctuations that can make her feel like she's on an emotional rollercoaster.

Your role is to be the lighthouse in the storm, offering a steady glow of empathy and understanding. It's about listening without judgment, comforting without offering unsolicited advice, and validating her feelings without trying to fix them. It's about understanding that this is a time of immense change for your partner, and what she needs most is your empathy and understanding.

Respecting the Healing Process

Now, imagine you're at a construction site, watching a building slowly rise, brick by brick, day by day. That's a little bit of what your partner's healing process looks like. It's slow, it's steady, and it requires patience.

Your partner's body has gone through the extraordinary experience of pregnancy and childbirth. It's going to take time to heal, to regain strength, and to adjust to the post-pregnancy state. It's important to respect this process and understand that it won't happen overnight.

Avoid putting pressure on her to "bounce back" or "get back to normal." Remember, this is a time of healing, of rest, and of adjustment. It's about helping her listen to her body, respect its signals, and give it the time it needs to recover.

Nurture Your Relationship During This Transition

Finally, let's talk about your relationship. It's like a garden that needs constant care and attention. And just like gardeners need to adjust their care routine with the changing seasons, you need to adjust your relationship care routine during this postpartum period.

Alright, new dads, let's approach post-baby intimacy like a well-crafted dish—timing is key, and a bit of patience adds to the flavor. While the six-week checkup is like the chef's recommendation, the real secret sauce is understanding. Your partner takes the lead in their recovery kitchen, and you're the supportive sous-chef awaiting the cue.

Imagine you and your partner starring in your own post-baby love story. The plot? Finding the perfect moment for a romantic scene. Remember, patience isn't just a virtue; it's the essential ingredient that shapes the narrative. So, sit back, enjoy the story, and consult with your healthcare provider for the best postpartum intimacy tips. They're the directors here—you're just part of the unfolding drama!

Recognize that your relationship is going through a transition. It's evolving from being a couple to being parents. This transition can bring new challenges, but it can also deepen your connection and bring you closer together.

Make time for each other. It could be a quiet chat after the baby is asleep, a shared laugh over a diaper change gone hilariously wrong, or a simple hug in the midst of a hectic day. These small moments of connection can nurture your relationship and help you navigate this transition together.

All in all, patience and understanding are key to supporting your partner during her postpartum recovery. Remember, you're her ally, her partner, her support system. Your patience can give her the space to heal, your understanding can lighten her emotional load, and your empathy can make her feel seen, heard, and valued. You're not just helping her recover; you're also strengthening your relationship and stepping into your role as a supportive partner and a loving dad.

As we wind down, remember this: Every act of patience, every gesture of understanding, every moment of empathy—they're all threads in the tapestry of your journey into fatherhood. Each thread strengthens the tapestry, adding color, depth, and resilience. So, hold on to these threads as we move forward, for they're not just threads; they're lifelines, guiding you, supporting you, and connecting you to your partner, your baby, and the incredible adventure of becoming a dad.

Chapter 10:

Breastfeeding 101—A Dad's Guide

Let's take a moment and picture a scene from a classic black-and-white movie. There's a hero, always ready to save the day, jumping into action at a moment's notice. Now, replace that hero with a modern-day superhero, you, the soon-to-be dad, and the action scene with a more serene setting—a quiet, cozy corner at home where your partner is breastfeeding your baby. This chapter, dear reader, is your training montage, preparing you to step into your role as a supportive partner during the breastfeeding journey.

The Basics of Breastfeeding: What Dads Should Know

Understanding the Breastfeeding Process

Breastfeeding is like a beautifully choreographed dance between the mother and baby. It begins with the 'latch,' where the baby attaches their mouth to the mother's breast, specifically the area around the nipple known as the areola. This latch triggers the release of two key hormones—prolactin and oxytocin.

Prolactin, the maestro of milk production, signals the mother's body to produce breast milk. It's like an orchestra conductor, ensuring each instrument (in this case, the milk-producing glands) is playing its part. Prolactin signals the body to produce breast milk, while oxytocin aids in milk delivery through the 'let-down' reflex (Mayo Clinic Health System, 2021; CDC, n.d.).

Oxytocin signals the muscles around the milk-producing glands to contract and push the milk towards the nipple, a process known as the 'let-down' reflex. It's akin to a relay race, where the baton (breast milk) is passed smoothly from one runner (milk duct) to another until it reaches the finish line (baby).

Benefits of Breastfeeding for Baby and Mom

Breastfeeding carries a host of benefits, both for the baby and the mom. It's like nature's all-in-one meal and medicine for the baby. Breast milk provides the perfect blend of nutrients that the baby needs for growth and development. It's also packed with antibodies that help protect the baby from various illnesses. Some studies even say it can make babies smarter! Infants who are breastfed typically experience fewer illnesses, reducing the likelihood of serious concerns such as Sudden Infant Death Syndrome (SIDS).

For the mom, breastfeeding can be a beautiful bonding experience with the baby. It's like their exclusive cuddle time, filled with warmth, love, and connection. It helps their bodies bounce back after having a baby by releasing a special hormone called oxytocin. Breastfeeding helps in post-pregnancy recovery and reduces the risk of certain cancers (Mayo Clinic Health System, 2021). It can also delay the return of menstrual periods, which is nature's way of ensuring some spacing between pregnancies. Moms who breastfeed have a smaller chance of getting certain cancers, like breast and ovarian cancers. It can even work as a kind of natural birth control in the beginning.

And guess what? Breastfeeding is super easy and saves money. There is no need for fancy bottles or clean-up—just mom and baby bonding time. It's good for the environment, too, because there's less stuff to make and throw away. But, you know what? Every family is different, and some moms choose other ways to feed their babies. What's most important is that everyone is happy and healthy!

Recognizing Common Breastfeeding Positions

Just like finding the most comfortable position to watch a movie marathon, discovering the optimal breastfeeding position is all about comfort—for both the mom and the baby. Common breastfeeding positions include the Cradle Hold, Cross-Cradle Hold, Football Hold, and Side-Lying Position. Each has its own comfort benefits and can be adapted to fit individual needs (Children's Hospital of Philadelphia, n.d.).

- **cradle hold**: The mom supports the baby's head in the crook of her arm. It's like cradling a football but a lot softer and sweeter.

- **cross cradle hold**: Similar to the cradle hold, the mom uses the opposite arm to support the baby. It's like doing the 'Heisman Trophy' pose but with a baby instead of a football.

- **football hold**: The baby's body is tucked under the mom's arm. It's a great position for moms who've had a C-section, as it keeps the baby's weight off the belly.

- **side-lying position**: The mom and the baby lie on their sides, facing each other. It's a comfortable position for moms who want to rest while breastfeeding.

Remember, every mom-baby duo is unique, and what works for one might not work for another. Encourage your partner to try different positions and see what's most comfortable for her and the baby. After all, breastfeeding is a journey of discovery, a dance, and finding the perfect rhythm can take some time and practice.

Well, future dad, that's the quick rundown on the basics of breastfeeding! Remember, knowledge is power. The more you understand about breastfeeding, the better you can support your partner in her journey. So, keep learning, keep asking questions, and keep being the amazing, supportive partner that you are. Because you're more than just watching from the sidelines; you're actively involved, a strong support, and an essential part of this breastfeeding journey.

The Breastfeeding Dojo: How to Be a Breastfeeding Ally

Offering Emotional Support

Picture yourself as a coach, standing on the sidelines during a critical game, cheering on your star player. That's the role you'll play as your partner navigates her breastfeeding quest.

Your cheers of encouragement, your high-fives of validation, your pats on the back of reassurance—they're all key ingredients in the recipe for emotional support.

Telling your partner that she's doing a great job, even when she's faced with challenges, can be a tremendous morale booster. Validate her efforts, empathize with her struggles, and celebrate her victories, no matter how small they seem.

Remember, it's not about solving problems or fixing things for her. It's about being there, listening, and reminding her of her strength and determination.

Assisting With Baby Positioning

Now, think of yourself as a choreographer, guiding your lead dancers into the perfect position for their performance. One of your roles in the breastfeeding dojo is to assist with baby positioning.

Helping your partner get comfortable and ensuring the baby is correctly positioned can make a world of difference during breastfeeding.

You can help by setting up pillows, assisting in positioning the baby, or gently guiding the baby's mouth toward the nipple. Remember, each session might require different adjustments (Children's Hospital of Philadelphia, n.d.). Think of it as strategically placing chess pieces on the board, making sure everything is in the right spot for the game to go smoothly. Additionally, when using a breastfeeding cover, be sure to hold it securely for the ultimate coverage of your partner's boobs or "private twins."

Keep in mind that each breastfeeding session might require different adjustments, and what worked once might not work the next time. So, stay adaptable, keep experimenting, and remember—your role is to assist, not direct.

Ensuring Mom's Comfort During Feeding

Finally, imagine you're a maître d' at a fancy restaurant, ensuring your patrons are comfortable and have everything they need for an enjoyable dining experience. That's a little bit of what ensuring mom's comfort during feeding is like.

You could bring her a glass of water or a healthy snack, offer to adjust her pillows, or provide a footrest to elevate her legs. Little acts of care like these can significantly enhance her comfort during feeding sessions.

Beyond physical comfort, consider her emotional comfort as well. Be there for her, listen, and share in the joy of these intimate moments with your baby.

So, future dad, are you ready to step into your breastfeeding dojo? Remember, your role is crucial. From offering emotional support to assisting with baby positioning and ensuring mom's comfort during feeding, each action, each gesture, and each word plays a part in this breastfeeding quest. So, step onto the mat, bow to your partner—your star player—and let's get this breastfeeding quest started. You're not just a spectator; you're an involved member, a crucial ally, and a key player in this quest. So, give it your all because this quest deserves nothing less.

The Breastfeeding Roadblocks: Navigating Common Challenges

Spotting Signs of a Poor Latch

Imagine driving a car with the seatbelt not properly buckled. It's there, but it's not providing the safety it's designed to. This is what a poor latch during breastfeeding can look like. The baby is attached to the breast, but not in the optimal way for effective feeding.

A proper latch involves the baby covering both the nipple and a substantial part of the areola, with their lips turned outward like a fish. It should be a comfortable experience for the mother. Spotting Signs of a Poor Latch: Look for signs like wincing in pain beyond the initial latch, a flat or pinched nipple after feeding, or the baby coming off the breast repeatedly (Children's Hospital of Philadelphia, n.d.).

Other clues include a clicking sound or the nipple looking flat or pinched after feeding. These are like warning lights on a car dashboard, signaling that something needs attention.

Unraveling Common Breastfeeding Issues Like Mastitis

Now, let's talk about a common speed bump on the breastfeeding route: mastitis. Picture a bustling city road suddenly blocked by a traffic jam.

Mastitis involves breast tissue inflammation, causing pain, swelling, and flu-like symptoms. Gentle massage and warm compresses can provide relief (Mayo Clinic Health System, 2021).

Blocked milk ducts frequently lead to mastitis. If a small amount of milk remains in the breast after feeds, it can block one of the milk ducts, causing it to become inflamed. It's like having a roadblock that disrupts the smooth flow of traffic.

While mastitis can be painful, it's essential to keep breastfeeding or pumping to help clear the blockage. Relief can be achieved by gently massaging the affected area and applying warm compresses.

Knowing When to Seek Professional Help

Imagine you're on a road trip, and suddenly, your car breaks down. You've tried everything you know, but it just won't start. What do you do? You call in a professional mechanic. Similarly, there are times on the breastfeeding journey when professional help might be needed.

If your partner is experiencing persistent pain during breastfeeding, if you suspect a poor latch that isn't improving, or if symptoms of mastitis don't start to improve within a few hours of home treatment, it's time to seek professional help. A lactation consultant, a healthcare professional specializing in breastfeeding, can provide invaluable support and advice.

Like a reliable roadside assistance service, these professionals can help troubleshoot the issues, provide practical help, and guide your partner toward a more comfortable and successful breastfeeding experience.

Navigating the breastfeeding road can have its challenges. But remember, every roadblock is an opportunity to learn, to grow, and to become a more confident and supportive partner. So, hold the map steady, keep the fuel of patience and understanding topped up, and continue on this breastfeeding ride. You're not just a passenger; you're a co-driver, navigating the breastfeeding challenges with your partner, one mile at a time.

Stepping Into the Spotlight: Dads in the Breastfeeding Arena

The Midnight Marathon: Assisting With Night Feedings

Picture an all-nighter, not the kind filled with pizza and video games, but one that involves soothing a hungry baby and sleep deprivation. Welcome, future dad, to the world of night feedings. This is a realm where time blurs, where moonlight becomes your companion, and where the soft coos of your baby become the soundtrack.

If your partner is breastfeeding, you might feel like a sidelined spectator during these night feedings. But guess what? You can be a part of this midnight marathon. If your baby is being bottle-fed, either with expressed breast milk or formula, take turns with your partner to handle the feedings. It's like tag-teaming in a relay race, sharing the load, and grabbing some extra sleep when off-duty.

Even if your partner is exclusively breastfeeding, there's plenty you can do. From changing diapers and burping the baby after feeds to rocking them back to sleep, you can be the supporting actor who adds depth to the scene.

Hydration and Nutrition: The Backstage Crew

Now, let's talk about the unsung heroes of the breastfeeding process—hydration and nutrition. They're like the backstage crew in a theater production, often overlooked but crucial for a successful performance.

Breastfeeding can make your partner thirsty and increase her need for fluids. Be her personal waterboy, keeping a bottle of water within her reach during feeds. A well-hydrated mom means a well-hydrated baby, so consider this your mission, should you choose to accept it.

Nutrition plays a vital role, too. Breastfeeding demands extra calories, and a balanced, nutritious diet is essential to ensure your partner has the energy she needs. Plus, here's the magic: what mom eats, so does the baby. It's like killing two birds with one stone—when the mom is eating healthy, the baby benefits, too. Ensure your partner stays hydrated and eats a nutritious diet to support breastfeeding (CDC, n.d.). You can play a role here by preparing healthy snacks for her to munch on during feeds or taking charge of meal preparation to ensure she's getting a mix of protein, carbohydrates, and fats in her diet. It's a win-win for both mom and the little one!

The Cheerleader: Offering Encouragement and Reassurance

Finally, consider yourself the cheerleader in your partner's breastfeeding journey. Your words of encouragement and reassurance can boost her confidence and lighten her emotional load.

Breastfeeding can be challenging, and there may be times when your partner feels overwhelmed or doubts her abilities. This is where your cheerleading skills come into play. An appreciative word about how she's doing a great job, a hug after a tough feeding session, or a simple 'You've got this!' can make her day.

Remember, your role is not to solve problems or provide solutions but to stand by her, offering your unwavering support and belief in her abilities.

And that's the scoop. Whether it's helping with night feedings, making sure your partner stays hydrated and well-fed, or being her biggest cheerleader, you're not merely watching from the sidelines in the breastfeeding journey; you're right in the thick of it, playing an active role. Each diaper changed, each glass of water fetched, and each word of encouragement is a testament to your role as a supportive partner and an involved dad. So, step into your role with confidence because you're about to make a world of difference in your partner's breastfeeding journey.

As we close this chapter, remember that the journey of fatherhood is not a solo expedition but a shared adventure. Every step you take, every role you play, every challenge you overcome brings you closer to becoming the dad you're meant to be. And as we turn the page, we'll explore another aspect of this adventure—balancing work responsibilities with fatherhood. So stay tuned, dear reader, because the adventure is just getting started.

Chapter 11:

Juggling Jobs: From Boardroom to Baby Room

Imagine walking a tightrope. On one side, you have your career, a realm filled with deadlines, meetings, and ambitions. On the other side, you have your family, a world brimming with first steps, bedtime stories, and unconditional love. As a new dad, you're that tightrope walker striving to maintain a delicate balance between work and family. But here's the good news—you don't have to do this balancing act alone. I'm here to share some practical tips and real-life strategies and, perhaps, play the role of your safety net as you navigate this high-wire work-life balance act. Ready to take the first step? Let's go!

The Challenge of Work-Life Balance

Adjusting to New Routines

Your alarm clock is no longer the buzz on your nightstand but the coos and cries of your little one. Your power suit has been replaced by a comfy t-shirt splashed with baby drool. And your carefully planned schedule? Well, that's now dictated by feeding times, diaper changes, and nap schedules.

Welcome to the new normal, where predictability is a thing of the past, and adaptability is the order of the day. Adjusting to these new routines can be challenging, but it's all part of the fatherhood package and crucial to finding a balance that works for you and your family (FatherResource, 2023). So, take a deep breath, embrace the unpredictability, and remember—this phase of sleepless nights and hectic days is temporary.

Managing Stress and Fatigue

Remember pulling all-nighters in college? The constant yawns, the heavy eyelids, the brain fog. Now, add to that the stress of diaper changes, colicky cries, and the overwhelming responsibility of caring for a tiny human. That's a glimpse into the life of a new dad.

Stress and fatigue are common, but they don't have to be your constant companions. Simple strategies like taking short power naps, practicing deep breathing exercises, or even stepping outside for a quick walk can help manage stress levels and combat fatigue (Workopolis, n.d.).

Prioritizing Family Time

Think back to your childhood. What are your fondest memories with your dad? Chances are, they're not extravagant vacations or expensive gifts but simple moments of connection—playing catch in the backyard, reading bedtime stories, or sharing pancakes on Sunday mornings.

Family time isn't about grand gestures; it's about being present, being involved, and creating memories. So, carve out time in your day to bond with your little one. It could be as simple as a morning cuddle, an afternoon stroll, or a lullaby before bedtime. It's these moments that turn everyday fatherhood into extraordinary memories.

As you juggle the demands of work and family, remember that it's not about achieving a perfect balance. It's about finding what works for you and your family, adjusting as needed, and giving yourself grace during this transition. You're not just a working professional; you're a dad. And that's a job title no boardroom can offer.

Practical Tips for Navigating Work and New Parenthood

Setting Boundaries at Work

Think of yourself as the ship's captain, navigating through the vast ocean of professional commitments while keeping a watchful eye on the distant shore of family life. The key to a smooth sail? Setting boundaries at work.

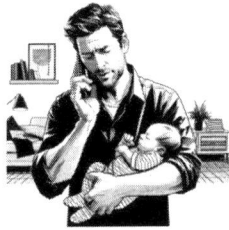

These boundaries protect your time, energy, and peace of mind like invisible guardrails. They can take many forms—a fixed cut-off time for checking emails, a 'no work on weekends' rule, or a clear communication to your team about your availability (FatherResource, 2023).

It's okay to switch off your work mode when you're at home. It's okay to say no to that late-night conference call or that weekend meeting. Remember, work is a part of your life, not your entire life. So, set those boundaries and ensure your ship sails smoothly between the world of work and the joy of fatherhood.

Utilizing Time Management Strategies

Picture yourself as a wizard with the power to control time. Sounds cool, right? While you may not have a magic wand, effective time management strategies can give you a semblance of this power.

Start by prioritizing your tasks. Not all work tasks are created equal, and understanding this can save you a lot of time and stress. Tackle high-priority tasks when your energy levels are at their peak, and save low-priority tasks for when you're winding down.

Next, consider batching similar tasks together. It's like doing laundry—you wouldn't wash one sock at a time, would you? Similarly, group and tackle similar work tasks in one focused time slot.

Lastly, don't underestimate the power of delegation. This helps in working smarter, not harder (Workopolis, n.d.). Assign tasks to others if they can complete them at least 80% as effectively. It's about working smarter, not harder.

Remember, time is a finite resource, but you can make the most of it with effective management. So, don your wizard hat and take control of your time, creating a work-life balance that suits you and your new role as a dad.

Seeking Support From Colleagues and Superiors

Now, imagine yourself as part of a relay race team. You're running your best race, but you know that your teammates are there, ready to take the baton when you need a breather. That's the kind of support you should seek from your colleagues and superiors at work.

Don't shy away from expressing your needs. Be open about your new responsibilities as a dad and the flexibility you might require. You'll be surprised how understanding and supportive your workmates can be.

Also, consider seeking a mentor, someone who's been in your shoes and can guide you through this transitional phase. Drawing from their experience can offer valuable insights and help you steer clear of common pitfalls.

Remember, you're not alone in this race. You're part of a team, both at work and at home. So, reach out, seek support, and remember, every relay race is won by teamwork, not individual effort. With the right support system at work, you can excel in your career without compromising on your responsibilities as a dad.

How to Advocate for Your Family at Work

Understanding Your Rights as a New Parent

Picture yourself at the helm of a ship, navigating through the choppy waters of parental rights. To steer your ship safely, you need a clear understanding of these rights. This includes the right to paternity leave, flexible working hours, and time off for family emergencies (FatherResource, 2023). In essence, you need to become well-versed with the laws and policies in your country and workplace that safeguard the interests of new parents.

This could include the right to paternity leave, the right to request flexible working hours, and the right to time off for family emergencies. It's like having a compass that guides you through the complexities of workplace policies, pointing you toward the provisions that support your new role as a dad.

So, take the time to learn about these rights. Reach out to your human resources department, consult your employment contract, and familiarize yourself with relevant labor laws. Remember, knowledge is power, and in this case, it's the power to advocate effectively for your family at work.

Communicating Your Needs Effectively

Now, let's turn our attention to the art of communication. Think of yourself as a diplomat, representing the interests of a newly formed nation—your family. Your mission is to communicate these interests clearly, effectively, and assertively to the larger entity of your workplace.

Start by identifying your needs. Do you need to adjust your working hours to accommodate for daycare pick-ups and drop-offs? Do you need to work from home a few days a week to share childcare responsibilities? Or do you need to take breaks during the day for parental duties?

Once you've identified your needs, it's time to communicate them. Prepare for this conversation with your boss or HR representative and use 'I' statements to express your feelings (FatherResource, 2023). Be clear, direct, and respectful in presenting your needs. Use 'I' statements to express your feelings and avoid sounding confrontational or defensive. For example, say, "I feel stressed because I'm unable to balance my work and family responsibilities. I need to adjust my working hours to better manage these roles."

Effective communication involves not only the content of your message but also the way you express it. Be confident and assertive, but also be open to compromise. After all, you're not just advocating for your needs; you're also building bridges of understanding and cooperation.

Negotiating for Flexible Work Arrangements

And finally, let's explore the negotiation table. Think of yourself as a skilled negotiator, striking a deal that benefits not just you but also your employer. The deal in question? Flexible work arrangements.

Flexible work arrangements can take many forms—telecommuting, flextime, compressed workweek, job sharing, or part-time work. They're like different flavors of ice cream, each catering to different tastes and preferences.

When negotiating for flexible work arrangements, present a clear plan to your employer. Describe how the proposed arrangement will work, how it will affect your productivity, and how it can benefit the company. It's about finding a win-win solution, one that supports your role as a dad while also meeting the needs of your employer.

Also, be prepared for possible objections and have your counterarguments ready. If your boss is concerned about your availability during work hours, assure them of your commitment to maintaining open lines of communication and responsiveness.

Negotiating for flexible work arrangements is not just about getting what you want. It's about creating a work environment that respects and supports your family's responsibilities. Describe how the proposed arrangement will work and how it can benefit the company (FatherResource, 2023; Workopolis, n.d.). Because at the end of the day, you're not just an employee or a colleague; you're a dad, and that's a role that deserves understanding, flexibility, and respect.

You're not just navigating the work-life balance; you're also setting a precedent, paving the way for future dads in your workplace to enjoy the same rights and flexibility. So, keep advocating, keep negotiating, and keep striving for a workplace that respects and supports your role as a dad. Because you're not just fighting for your rights; you're also championing the rights of many others. And that's a cause worth fighting for.

Making the Most of Paternity Leave

Planning for Paternity Leave

Think of paternity leave as a well-deserved vacation. But instead of basking in the sun on a tropical beach, you're navigating the beautiful chaos of new parenthood. Even though it's different, planning for it is just as crucial.

Plan your paternity leave by understanding your company's policies and discussing your leave with your employer well in advance. This helps in making the most of this crucial time (FatherResource, 2023). How much time can you take off? Is it paid or unpaid? Can you split the leave into parts? Getting clarity on these questions is like mapping out your itinerary, ensuring you know exactly what lies ahead.

Next, discuss your leave with your employer well in advance. It's like booking your vacation tickets early to avoid last-minute hassles. This conversation also gives your employer ample time to plan for your temporary absence.

Maximizing Bonding Time With Baby

Now, let's talk about the heart of paternity leave—bonding with your baby. This is like the highlight of your vacation, the part you look forward to the most.

Savor simple moments, like cuddling your baby, making silly faces, or singing lullabies. These intimate interactions are like threads that weave the beautiful bond between you and your baby. Maximizing bonding time with your baby is central to paternity leave. Savor simple moments of connection, which are crucial in building a strong bond with your child (FatherResource, 2023).

Keep in mind that bonding is not solely determined by the amount of time spent together but also by the quality of that time. So, put away your phone, forget about your to-do list, and immerse yourself in the world of your little one. The most profound connections are made in these quiet, heartfelt moments.

Supporting Your Partner During Leave

During your paternity leave, another crucial role you'll play is that of your partner's support system. Think of yourself as the trusty sidekick, always ready to step in and lend a hand.

This could mean taking over diaper duty, preparing meals, or simply holding the baby while your partner takes a nap. Small acts of assistance can make a big difference in easing your partner's load.

But don't forget emotional support. Listen to your partner's concerns, validate her feelings, and offer words of encouragement. Your emotional support can be a beacon of strength for her during this transformative period.

As we wrap up this chapter, remember that balancing work and family life is not a one-time act but an ongoing process. It's about setting boundaries, managing your time effectively, advocating for your family, and making the most of your paternity leave. This delicate balancing act may seem daunting, but you'll find your rhythm with each passing day. You're not just juggling jobs; you're also building a life that cherishes both your professional ambitions and your beautiful new role as a dad. As we move forward, we'll explore more aspects of this incredible adventure and equip you with the tools and insights you need to navigate the path of fatherhood with confidence and joy. So, let's turn the page and see what the next chapter holds.

Chapter 12:

Strengthening Bonds—From Couplehood to Parenthood

Picture this: you and your partner are skilled dancers, moving in perfect sync, effortlessly gliding across the dance floor. Suddenly, the music changes. The rhythm is new, the melody unfamiliar. This is what transitioning from being a couple to becoming a parent can feel like. It's a shift in tune that requires you to learn new steps, change your rhythm, and sometimes, even stumble a bit. But here's the good news: together, you can learn to dance to this new melody and create a beautiful performance. So, lace up your dancing shoes, and let's get started.

Navigating Relationship Changes During Pregnancy and Beyond

Understanding Changes in Relationship Dynamics

Remember the time you and your partner decided to rearrange the furniture in your living room? It was challenging and sometimes frustrating, but eventually, you found a layout that worked. The transition to parenthood is a bit like that—it requires rearranging the dynamics of your relationship to accommodate a new addition.

Your roles expand from being partners to being co-parents. Your 'us' time might get replaced by 'family' time. Conversations can shift from discussing work or weekend plans to baby feeds and diaper changes. These changes are natural and expected. But understanding them can help you navigate through this transition smoothly (NCT, 2022).

Addressing Common Relationship Challenges Post-Baby

Think back to a time when you tried a complex recipe for the first time. It was probably fraught with challenges—missing ingredients, burnt edges, and perhaps even a kitchen disaster or two. Post-baby relationship challenges can feel a bit like that—overwhelming but not insurmountable.

One common challenge is the division of baby care responsibilities. As new parents, both of you are learning on the job, which can sometimes lead to disagreements or misunderstandings. It's like trying to assemble a piece of furniture without a manual.

Sometimes, exhaustion from sleepless nights and constant baby care can result in short tempers and heightened emotions. It's like operating on a low battery—even simple tasks feel challenging, and patience runs thin.

The key to addressing these challenges lies in open communication, mutual understanding, and shared problem-solving. It's about turning that complicated recipe into a teamwork exercise rather than a solo task (NCT, 2022; UCLA Health, 2022).

Fostering Mutual Respect and Understanding

Imagine yourself as a gardener, tending to the plants in your garden with care and patience. Fostering mutual respect and understanding in your relationship post-baby is a lot like that. It requires constant tending, a lot of patience, and a dash of love.

Respect each other's parenting style. Just like no two gardeners have the same technique, no two parents have the same parenting approach. Appreciate the unique strengths that each of you brings to the parenting table.

Understand that each parent bonds with the baby in their own way. It's like how sunflowers turn towards the sun, while ivy plants prefer the shade. Both are valid and beautiful in their own way.

Remember, you and your partner are on the same team. Like two gardeners tending to the same garden, you're both working towards the common goal of raising a happy, healthy child. Nurturing mutual respect and understanding can help your relationship flourish, even as you navigate the challenges of parenthood (NCT, 2022).

Chapter 12 is about understanding and navigating the changes in your relationship as you transition from being a couple to becoming parents. It's about tackling the challenges, fostering mutual respect and understanding, and learning to dance to the new melody of parenthood. So keep dancing, keep learning, and keep loving because the dance floor of parenthood is filled with surprises, joy, and a love like no other.

The Importance of Open Communication

Encouraging Honest Dialogue

Think of your relationship as a safe harbor, a place where honesty is the anchor that holds your ship steady. As new parents, encouraging honest dialogue is like maintaining that anchor, ensuring that your relationship remains stable amidst the changing tides of parenthood (NCT, 2022).

How do you cultivate this honesty? Imagine you're in a game of catch. You throw the ball, your partner catches it, and then throws it back. Similarly, in an honest dialogue, you express your thoughts, and your partner listens and then responds.

This back-and-forth exchange builds trust and openness, creating a safe space where both of you can share your feelings, fears, and hopes about parenthood. It's like polishing that anchor, keeping it strong and reliable, no matter how turbulent the seas get.

Expressing Feelings and Concerns Effectively

Now, let's take a moment to talk about expressing feelings and concerns. Picture yourself as a painter; your words are your colors, and your relationship is the canvas. The way you express your feelings and concerns can either create a beautiful masterpiece or a confusing jumble of colors.

The key to effective expression lies in being clear, concise, and considerate. It's about saying what you feel without blaming or criticizing your partner. It's about using 'I' statements instead of 'You' statements. For instance, say, "I feel overwhelmed when the baby cries, and I can't soothe them," instead of "You always hand over the baby when they're crying."

This method enables you to communicate your concerns without causing defensiveness in your partner. It's like choosing the right colors to create harmony on the canvas, making your feelings and concerns clear without causing discord in your relationship.

Listening Actively and Empathetically

Finally, let's flip the coin and look at the other side of communication—listening. Think of yourself as a mirror, reflecting your partner's words and emotions. Active and empathetic listening is about being that mirror, showing your partner that you understand and validate their feelings (UCLA Health, 2022).

Active listening entails giving your full attention to your partner, minimizing distractions, and responding appropriately. It's about giving them the space to express themselves without interrupting or imposing your views.

Empathetic listening goes a step further. It's about putting yourself in your partner's shoes and trying to understand their perspective. It's about validating their feelings, even if you don't necessarily agree with them. It's like angling the mirror so that it reflects your partner's emotions accurately and compassionately.

Creating an environment of open communication is like charting a clear course for your ship through the vast ocean of parenthood. By encouraging honest dialogue, expressing feelings and concerns effectively, and listening actively and empathetically, you and your partner can navigate this course together, weathering storms, enjoying calm seas, and cherishing the beautiful voyage that is parenthood.

Keeping the Romance Alive: Date Night Ideas for New Parents

Planning At-Home Date Nights

Imagine you're on a secret mission, transforming your living room into a cozy bistro, complete with candlelight, soft music, and a delicious meal. Welcome to the world of at-home date nights, where the ambiance is as comforting as the person across the table.

Planning at-home date nights is like unwrapping a gift that keeps on giving. It's about rediscovering the joy of each other's company amidst the baby bottles and diaper changes.

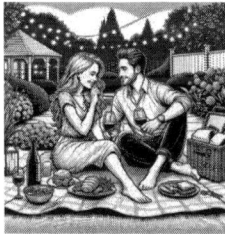

Start by setting the scene. It could be a romantic dinner at your dining table, a movie night in your living room, or a picnic in your backyard. The key is to create an atmosphere that's different from your daily routine. It's like stepping into a magic portal that transports you from the world of parenthood to the world of romance.

Next, plan an activity that both of you enjoy. It could be cooking a meal together, watching a movie, or simply talking about your dreams and aspirations. It's about reconnecting as a couple, reminding each other that beyond being parents, you're also partners (NCT, 2022).

Remember, at-home date nights aren't about extravagant gestures or elaborate plans. They're about creating pockets of 'us' time in the hurricane of 'family' time. They're about reminding each other that amidst the chaos of new parenthood, your love for each other remains unwavering.

Incorporating Small Gestures of Love Daily

Now, let's shift the spotlight to daily life. Think of it as a canvas, where small gestures of love are splashes of vibrant colors, adding warmth and beauty to the picture.

Incorporating small gestures of love into your daily routine is like sprinkling magic dust on an ordinary day. It's about showing love and appreciation in simple, heartfelt ways.

It could be as simple as making a cup of coffee for your partner in the morning, leaving a sweet note in their lunchbox, or giving them a foot massage after a long day. It's about taking a moment from your day to say 'I love you' in actions, not just words.

Remember, these small gestures might not seem like much, but they can make a big difference in keeping the romance alive. They're like gentle whispers of love, reminding your partner that they're cherished, appreciated, and loved.

Utilizing Family or Babysitter Support for Occasional Outings

Finally, let's venture outside the home. Imagine you're explorers embarking on an adventure, just the two of you. Welcome to the world of occasional outings, where the baby stays at home, and you get a few hours of couple time.

Occasional outings are like refreshing pit stops on the marathon of parenthood. They give you a chance to step out of your parenting roles and enjoy each other's company without interruptions or baby duties.

Start by arranging for a reliable babysitter or a family member to watch over the baby. It's like leaving your treasure in safe hands while you go on an adventure.

Next, plan an outing that both of you will enjoy. It could be a dinner at your favorite restaurant, a walk in the park, or a visit to a museum. The goal is to spend quality time together, away from the responsibilities of home (NCT, 2022).

Remember, occasional outings are not about escaping from parenthood. They're about reconnecting as a couple and recharging your batteries. They're about reminding each other that even though you're parents, you're also lovers, friends, and partners.

The Power of Teamwork in Parenting

Sharing Baby Care Responsibilities

Picture a doubles match in tennis. The key to winning isn't just about having the best individual players, but it's about how well they work as a team—coordinating movements, covering the court effectively, and playing to each other's strengths. The realm of parenting isn't all that different. It's about teaming up with your partner to tackle the game of baby care.

As new parents, the baby care duties might seem like a long rally of feeding, changing, burping, soothing, and repeating. Sharing these responsibilities can turn this rally into a well-coordinated play.

Maybe you're a pro at diapering, and your partner has the magic touch to soothe the baby. Perhaps your partner is a night owl, perfect for those late-night feeds, while you're an early bird, ready to take over in the morning. The key is to play to your strengths, divide the tasks, and step in for each other when needed. It's not just about making the game easier; it's also about enjoying the play and celebrating the little wins together.

Making Decisions Together

Now, imagine you're on a road trip. You and your partner are in the car, map in hand, deciding which routes to take, where to stop, and what sights to see. Parenting decisions are a lot like that roadmap. They're about charting the course of your baby's life, from small decisions like choosing a brand of baby food to bigger ones like selecting a school.

Making these decisions together is like navigating that roadmap as a team. It's about discussing options, weighing pros and cons, and reaching a consensus. It's about respecting each other's viewpoints, compromising when needed, and always keeping your baby's best interests at heart.

Remember, the goal isn't about who's right or who's wrong. It's about finding the best route for your baby, even if it means taking a few detours or making unexpected stops. After all, the joy of a road trip isn't just about reaching the destination; it's also about the shared experience of the journey (UCLA Health, 2022).

Supporting Each Other's Parenting Styles

Finally, let's think of parenting styles as different musical instruments. Your partner might be a piano, providing the steady rhythm and harmony, while you might be a guitar, adding the melody and flair. Both instruments are different, but when played together, they create beautiful music.

Supporting each other's parenting styles is about creating that symphony. It's about appreciating the unique tunes each of you brings to the parenting ensemble. It's about coordinating your rhythms, adjusting your volumes, and playing in harmony, even if your tunes are different.

Perhaps your partner is more structured in their approach, following schedules and routines, while you're more spontaneous, turning baby care into a fun game. Instead of trying to outplay each other, find ways to harmonize your styles (UCLA Health, 2022).

Remember, there's no one 'right' way to parent. Every style has its melody, every approach, and its rhythm. The key is to respect each other's tunes, support each other's solos, and always aim for harmony. Because together, you're not just playing random notes; you're creating a symphony of love, care, and nurturing for your baby.

And that wraps it up. Whether you're dividing baby care duties, jointly making decisions, or backing each other's parenting approaches, teamwork is the essential element that weaves everything together. It's about dancing to the new melody of parenthood, navigating the roadmap of decisions, and creating a symphony of harmonious parenting. So, keep playing, keep dancing, and keep loving because your teamwork is making the dream work. As we gear up for the next chapter, remember this: Parenthood isn't a solo performance; it's a duet—a beautiful, heartfelt duet that's best played together.

Keeping The Fatherhood Fun Rolling

Now that you've geared up with all the tips and tricks to embrace fatherhood, it's your turn to pass the baton and guide other soon-to-be dads toward this incredible resource.

By sharing your honest thoughts about "Ready, Set, Dad: A Complete Pregnancy Guide for Men" on Amazon, you're not just leaving a review. You're lighting the way for other dads-to-be, showing them where they can find the same support, laughter, and practical wisdom that you discovered.

Your voice matters. Every review and every shared experience helps keep the spirit of informed and joyful fatherhood alive. And by doing so, you're playing a crucial role in our mission at S. L. Diverson – to empower fathers everywhere.

So, take a moment and click the link below to leave your review on Amazon. It's more than just words; it's a beacon for the next dad, eagerly searching for guidance and a friendly voice in the world of fatherhood.

Scan the QR code to leave your review on Amazon.

Thank you for joining us on this journey. Your contribution keeps the joy and wisdom of fatherhood thriving, one review at a time.

With gratitude,

S. L. Diverson

Conclusion

Well, my friend, we've journeyed through the wild terrain of first-time fatherhood together, navigating morning sickness, diaper changes, and even the dreaded assembly of baby furniture. If you're still reading this, it either means you have successfully mastered the art of one-handed book-holding while bottle-feeding, or you've managed to hide in the bathroom long enough to finish this passage. Either way, kudos to you!

In our expedition, we've covered everything from understanding pregnancy (it's not just about the cravings, folks) and labor (no, not the one that involves fixing things around the house) to the art of swaddling (not to be mistaken with smuggling). We've dealt with the emotional rollercoaster (you thought it was just her hormones, didn't you?) and even tiptoed around the landmines of postpartum recovery (yes, she's still the woman you once knew, just a bit more...explosive).

The key takeaway? Embrace the chaos, my friend. Fatherhood is like trying to assemble a piece of IKEA furniture—it's confusing, the instructions are never clear, and you're always left with a nagging feeling that you've done something wrong. But in the end, the finished product is a beautiful, wobbly...I mean, sturdy masterpiece that you can't help but be proud of.

Remember, you're not just a "dad-in-training;" you're the emotional rock, the diaper-disposal hero, the master swaddler, and the carrier of all things baby-related. But most importantly, you're the co-star in the amazing parenthood journey. So, take a deep breath, strap on that baby carrier, and step confidently onto the stage.

And finally, a call to action. Laugh. Laugh at the spit-up on your last clean shirt, the 2 a.m. diaper explosions, and the fact that you now consider a six-hour sleep stretch a luxury. Laughter is the best tool you have to navigate the maze of fatherhood. Plus, it's a lot cheaper than therapy.

As we close the book (pun intended) on this fatherhood guide, remember that every dad, no matter how put-together he seems, has stood where you stand—a little confused, a lot overwhelmed, and wildly unprepared. But guess what? They made it through, and so will you.

So, here's to you, future dad. May your dad jokes always be corny, your baby's giggles infectious, and your journey into fatherhood filled with love, laughter, and an endless supply of wet wipes. Welcome to the Dad Club!

References

Agrawal, J., Chakole, S., & Sachdev, C. (2022). The Role of Fathers in Promoting Exclusive Breastfeeding. *Cureus*, *14*(10). https://doi.org/10.7759/cureus.30363

Allina Health. (n.d.). *Postpartum Emotions | Postpartum Depression.* Allinahealth.org.

American Academy of Pediatrics. (n.d.). *Building Your Support System.* Aap.org.

American Psychological Association. (n.d.). *Paternal Concerns and Challenges.* Apa.org.

APTA Pelvic Health. (2023). *Guiding the Journey: A Comprehensive Exploration of Postpartum Recovery for Physical Therapists.* Aptapelvichealth.org.

Australia, H. (2023, February 17). *A partner's guide to breastfeeding – how to help and support your partner.* Www.pregnancybirthbaby.org.au. https://www.pregnancybirthbaby.org.au/a-partners-guide-to-breastfeeding

Australian Parenting. (2023, July 12). *Raising children as a team: why it's important.* Raising Children Network. https://raisingchildren.net.au/grown-ups/looking-after-yourself/parenting/parenting-teamwork

Bellefonds, C. de. (2023, December 14). *17 Ways to Relieve Morning Sickness.* What to Expect. https://www.whattoexpect.com/pregnancy/morning-sickness/

Better Health Channel. (2018, May 25). *Pregnancy stages and changes.* Www.betterhealth.vic.gov.au. https://www.betterhealth.vic.gov.au/health/HealthyLiving/pregnancy-stages-and-changes

Boyd-Barrett, C. (2021). *Morning sickness during pregnancy | BabyCenter.* BabyCenter. https://www.babycenter.com/pregnancy/your-body/morning-sickness_254

Centers for Disease Control and Prevention (CDC). (n.d.). *Newborn Breastfeeding Basics.* Cdc.gov.

Children's Hospital of Philadelphia. (n.d.). *Breastfeeding Tips for Beginners.* Chop.edu.

Cleveland Clinic. (2023a). *A Guide To Childproofing Your Home.* Clevelandclinic.org.

Cleveland Clinic. (2023b, March 3). *Stages of pregnancy & fetal development | Cleveland clinic.* Cleveland Clinic. https://my.clevelandclinic.org/health/articles/7247-fetal-development-stages-of-growth

Coleman, P. A. (2018, March 1). *The 15 Things That Need to Get Done Before You Bring Home a Baby.* Fatherly. https://www.fatherly.com/parenting/dad-checklist-fathers-need-to-do-before-baby

Consumer Product Safety Commission. (n.d.). *Childproofing Your Home - Several Safety Devices to Help Protect Your Children from Home Hazards.* Cpsc.gov.

Dad Gold. (2021, August 18). *4 Easy Ways Dad Can Bond With His Unborn Baby - Dad Gold.* Dadgold.com. https://dadgold.com/how-dad-can-bond-with-unborn-baby/

Douglas, T. B. (2023, March). *4 Mistakes I've Made as a Man During My Partner's Pregnancy.* Good Man Project. https://goodmenproject.com/featured-content/4-mistakes-ive-made-as-a-man-during-my-partners-pregnancy/

Eldemire, A. (2017, January 23). *The One Conversation That New Parents Need to Stay Connected.* The Gottman Institute. https://www.gottman.com/blog/one-conversation-new-parents-need-stay-connected/

Fatherly. (n.d.). *Benefits of Dad Support Groups.* Fatherly.com.

FatherResource. (2023). *What Will the Future of Work-Life Balance Look Like for Fathers?* Fatherresource.org.

Forbes. (n.d.). *Financial Planning for New Parents.* Forbes.com.

Franzen, J., Cornet, I., Vendittelli, F., & Guittier, M.-J. (2021). First-time fathers' experience of childbirth: a cross-sectional study. *Midwifery, 103,* 103153. https://doi.org/10.1016/j.midw.2021.103153

Galla, S. (n.d.). *Father Support Groups - A Guide to Support Groups for Dads [2020].* MensGroup.com. Retrieved December 20, 2023, from https://mensgroup.com/father-support-groups/

Garfield, C. (n.d.). *FATHERS, PREGNANCY AND THE PERINATAL PERIOD.* https://www.nichd.nih.gov/sites/default/files/about/meetings/2015/Documents/3-Garfield-Fathers_Pregnancy.pdf

Garvey, M. (2022, January 21). *15 At-Home Date Night Ideas for New Parents.* Www.thebump.com. https://www.thebump.com/a/at-home-date-night-ideas-for-parents

Giurgescu, C., & Templin, T. N. (2015). Father Involvement and Psychological Well-Being of Pregnant Women. *MCN, the American Journal of Maternal/Child Nursing, 40*(6), 381–387. https://doi.org/10.1097/nmc.0000000000000183

Gruber, K. J., Cupito, S. H., & Dobson, C. F. (2013). Impact of Doulas on Healthy Birth Outcomes. *The Journal of Perinatal Education, 22*(1), 49–58. https://doi.org/10.1891/1058-1243.22.1.49

Harvard Business Review. (n.d.). *Work-Life Balance for Parents.* Hbr.org.

Headspace. (n.d.). *Benefits of Mindfulness.* Headspace.com.

Healthline. (n.d.). *Exercise and Stress Management.* Healthline.com.

Healthy relationships with partners in pregnancy. (2022, November 10). Raising Children Network. https://raisingchildren.net.au/pregnancy/pregnancy-for-partners/relationships-and-feelings/healthy-relationships-with-partners-pregnancy

Horizons, B. (2021, July 15). *Pregnancy for Dads: A Father's Role before the Baby Arrives.* Www.brighthorizons.com. https://www.brighthorizons.com/resources/Article/Pregnancy-for-Dads-A-Fathers-Role-before-the-Baby-Arrives

How do I assemble and install baby furniture safely? (2023, June 18). WakeUpDeals.com. https://wakeupdeals.com/listing/how-do-i-assemble-and-install-baby-furniture-safely/

How Parents Can Instill a Growth Mindset at Home. (2017). Mindsetworks.com. https://www.mindsetworks.com/parents/growth-mindset-parenting

Johns Hopkins Medicine. (n.d.). *Baby Blues and Postpartum Depression: Mood Disorders and Pregnancy.* Hopkinsmedicine.org.

Johns Hopkins Medicine. (2019). *Hormones During Pregnancy.* Johns Hopkins Medicine. https://www.hopkinsmedicine.org/health/conditions-and-diseases/staying-healthy-during-pregnancy/hormones-during-pregnancy

Johnson, C. (2018, January 29). *Morning Sickness Survival Kit.* Life with My Littles. https://www.lifewithmylittles.com/morning-sickness-survival-kit/

Kessler, O. (2023, December 4). *Empathic Listening in Relationships: Meaning, Examples, and Tips.* Marriage Advice - Expert Marriage Tips & Advice. https://www.marriage.com/advice/relationship/empathic-listening/

Lawrence, T. E. (2021, May 24). *Reading To Your Baby During Pregnancy Is Worth The Book Club With Your Belly Button.* Romper. https://www.romper.com/pregnancy/the-benefits-of-reading-to-your-baby-during-pregnancy-experts

Le Page, M. (2023, June 8). *We finally know what causes morning sickness during pregnancy.* NewScientist. https://www.newscientist.com/article/2377397-we-finally-know-what-causes-morning-sickness-during-pregnancy/

MacDonald, E. (2018, May 17). *First Trimester Pregnancy Guide For Dads.* My Baby's Heartbeat Bear. https://www.mybabysheartbeatbear.com/blogs/pregnancy/first-trimester-pregnancy-guide-for-the-expecting-fathers

Manual, B. (2018, March 27). *Vaginal Birth vs. C-Section: Pros & Cons.* Live Science; Live Science. https://www.livescience.com/45681-vaginal-birth-vs-c-section.html

Masters, M. (2021, November 5). *A Partner's Guide to Life After Childbirth.* What to Expect. https://www.whattoexpect.com/pregnancy/for-dad/life-after-childbirth.aspx

Mayo Clinic. (n.d.). *Pregnancy week by week.* Mayo Clinic. https://www.mayoclinic.org/healthy-lifestyle/pregnancy-week-by-week/in-depth/prenatal-care/art-20044581

Mayo Clinic. (2018). *Postpartum care: After a vaginal delivery*. Mayo Clinic. https://www.mayoclinic.org/healthy-lifestyle/labor-and-delivery/in-depth/postpartum-care/art-20047233

Mayo Clinic. (2020, June 30). *Fetal development: What happens during the 3rd trimester?* Mayo Clinic. https://www.mayoclinic.org/healthy-lifestyle/pregnancy-week-by-week/in-depth/fetal-development/art-20045997

Mayo Clinic. (2021). *Breastfeeding 101: Tips for new moms*. Mayoclinichealthsystem.org.

Mayo Clinic. (2022a, January 13). *Stages of Labor and birth: Baby, it's time!* Mayo Clinic. https://www.mayoclinic.org/healthy-lifestyle/labor-and-delivery/in-depth/stages-of-labor/art-20046545

Mayo Clinic. (2022b, September 28). *Morning sickness - Diagnosis and treatment - Mayo Clinic*. Www.mayoclinic.org. https://www.mayoclinic.org/diseases-conditions/morning-sickness/diagnosis-treatment/drc-20375260

Mayo Clinic. (2022c, November 24). *Postpartum depression - diagnosis and treatment*. Mayoclinic.org. https://www.mayoclinic.org/diseases-conditions/postpartum-depression/diagnosis-treatment/drc-20376623

McConnell, L. (2022, September 14). *8 (Realistic) Ways Working Dads Can Achieve Work-Life Balance | Ivy Exec*. Ivyexec.com. https://ivyexec.com/career-advice/2022/8-realistic-ways-working-dads-can-achieve-work-life-balance

Melissa, & Doug. (2023, November 20). *3 Brain-Building Ways to Play With Your Baby*. HealthyChildren.org. https://www.healthychildren.org/English/family-life/power-of-play/Pages/brain-building-ways-to-play-with-your-baby.aspx?_gl=1

Mental Health America. (n.d.). *Seeking Professional Help*. Mhanational.org.

MindTools. (n.d.). *Visualization Techniques*. Mindtools.com.

MountainStar Medical Group. (2023, November 2). *A partner's guide to supporting women's health during pregnancy*. KSL.com. https://www.ksl.com/article/50493857/a-partners-guide-to-supporting-womens-health-during-pregnancy

Murray, RN, BSN, D. (2020, April 20). *Common Breastfeeding Problems and How to Deal With Them*. Verywell Family. https://www.verywellfamily.com/common-problems-of-breastfeeding-431906

National Institutes of Health. (n.d.). *Importance of Social Support*. Nih.gov.

National Safety Council. (n.d.). *Childproofing*. Nsc.org.

NHS. (2020, December 2). *Tips for your birth partner*. Nhs.uk. https://www.nhs.uk/pregnancy/labour-and-birth/what-happens/tips-for-your-birth-partner/

Parenting Magazine. (n.d.). *Embracing Fatherhood*. Parenting.com.

Physical and Emotional Changes During Pregnancy | babyMed.com. (2009, May 6). *Physical and Emotional Changes During Pregnancy | babyMed.com*. BabyMed.com. https://www.babymed.com/pregnancy/physical-and-emotional-changes-during-pregnancy

Popper, N. (2020, April 17). Paternity Leave Has Long-Lasting Benefits. So Why Don't More American Men Take It? *The New York Times*. https://www.nytimes.com/2020/04/17/parenting/paternity-leave.html

Positive Psychology. (n.d.). *Psychological Benefits of Daily Affirmations*. Positivepsychology.com.

Pregnancy and Mental Health. (n.d.). Center for Neuroscience in Women's Health. https://med.stanford.edu/womensneuroscience/wellness_clinic/Pregnancy.html

pregnancy-role-of-the-father-to-be. (2023, November 22). Www.healthhub.sg. https://www.healthhub.sg/live-healthy/pregnancy-role-of-the-father-to-be

PsychCentral. (n.d.). *Impact of Celebrating Small Wins*. Psychcentral.com.

Psychology Today. (n.d.). *Fear of the Unknown*. Psychologytoday.com.

Ruitenburg, H., van den Berg, S. W., & Garssen, J. (2021). *The role of the partner in the support of a pregnant woman's healthy diet: an explorative qualitative study*. BMC Pregnancy and Childbirth. https://bmcpregnancychildbirth.biomedcentral.com/articles/10.1186/s12884-021-04027-2

S., A., R.S., B., & L., G. (2021). *Women's experiences of social support during pregnancy: a qualitative systematic review*. BMC Pregnancy and Childbirth. https://bmcpregnancychildbirth.biomedcentral.com/articles/10.1186/s12884-021-03746-w

Sangster, M. (n.d.). *Hospital Bag Checklist For Dad: 18 Must-Have Items*. Nanit. https://www.nanit.com/blogs/parent-confidently/hospital-bag-checklist

Services, D. of H. & H. (2023, June 18). *Pregnancy support - fathers, partners and carers*. Www.betterhealth.vic.gov.au. https://www.betterhealth.vic.gov.au/health/servicesandsupport/pregnancy-support-fathers-partners-and-carers

Sihota, H., Oliffe, J., Kelly, M. T., & McCuaig, F. (2019). Fathers' Experiences and Perspectives of Breastfeeding: A Scoping Review. *American Journal of Men's Health*, *13*(3), 155798831985161. https://doi.org/10.1177/1557988319851616

Smithurst, B. (2021, September 15). *What Dads Can Expect in the 2nd Trimester - Huggies*. Www.huggies.com.au. https://www.huggies.com.au/parenting/dads-journey/dad-expects-pregnancy-second-trimester

Sparks, D. (2021, June 17). *New dad: Tips to help manage stress.* Mayo Clinic News Network. https://newsnetwork.mayoclinic.org/discussion/new-dad-tips-to-help-manage-stress/

The Bump. (n.d.). *New Dads Groups and Their Benefits.* Thebump.com.

The Bump Editors. (2014, September 19). *Your Ultimate Baby Proofing Checklist.* Thebump.com; The Bump. https://www.thebump.com/a/checklist-babyproofing-part-1

The Gottman Institute. (n.d.). *Open Communication in Relationships.* Gottman.com.

The Mother Baby Center. (n.d.). *What to expect during the postpartum recovery period.* Themotherbabycenter.org.

Tommy's. (n.d.). *Your partner's emotions during pregnancy - for dads and partners.* Tommy's. https://www.tommys.org/pregnancy-information/im-pregnant/pregnancy-calendar/second-trimester-weeks-13-27/your-partners-emotions-during-pregnancy-dads-and-partners

Trifu, S., Vladuti, A., & Popescu, A. (2019). Neuroendocrine Aspects of Pregnancy and Postpartum Depression. *Acta Endocrinologica (Bucharest), 15*(3), 410–415. https://doi.org/10.4183/aeb.2019.410

Trust), N. (National C. (2019, April 2). *Dad-to-be guide: 10 facts for the third trimester.* NCT (National Childbirth Trust). https://www.nct.org.uk/pregnancy/dads-be/dad-be-guide-10-facts-for-third-trimester

U.S. Department of Health & Human Services. (2016, December 13). *Body changes and discomforts | womenshealth.gov.* Womenshealth.gov. https://www.womenshealth.gov/pregnancy/youre-pregnant-now-what/body-changes-and-discomforts

Understand parental leave and your employer obligations. (2023, November 1). Australia. https://employmenthero.com/resources/understanding-parental-leave/

Valiani, M., & HadiAlijanvand, S. (2021). The Effect of Fetus Stimulation Techniques on Newborn Behavior. *Iranian Journal of Nursing and Midwifery Research, 26*(6), 550–554. https://doi.org/10.4103/ijnmr.IJNMR_142_20

Vanderkam, L. (2020, April 18). *Have a Baby and Still Want to Get Things Done?* Nytimes.com; The New York Times. https://www.nytimes.com/article/new-parents-time-management-guide.html

Watson, S. (2023, March 3). *Fetal Movement: Feeling the Baby Kick.* WebMD. https://www.webmd.com/baby/fetal-movement-feeling-baby-kick

What Your Partner Should Know About the First Trimester. (2022). Lancastergeneralhealth.org. https://www.lancastergeneralhealth.org/health-hub-home/motherhood/your-pregnancy/what-your-partner-should-know-about-the-first-trimester

Workopolis. (n.d.). *5 work-life balance tips for new working dads.* Careers.workopolis.com.

Wu Ph.D., K. (2020, December 27). *Top 17 Fears of New Fathers During Pregnancy | Psychology Today.* Www.psychologytoday.com. https://www.psychologytoday.com/us/blog/the-modern-heart/202012/top-17-fears-new-fathers-during-pregnancy

Printed in Great Britain
by Amazon

51467549R00079